Praise for *Sacred Sound*

"Alanna Kaivalya bravely tackles the subtlest, most elusive of all spiritual methods: the power of sound — compelling vibrations conveyed to our innermost selves through ancient mantra. Then she adds layers of meaning by laying out the fascinating mythic stories at their core. It's an inspiring and potent potion for spiritual growth."

— Jack Hawley, author of the award-winning *Bhagavad Gita: A Walkthrough for Westerners*

"Alanna Kaivalya is a storyteller, bard, and great teacher, using mythology and mantra to reintroduce us to deep basic truths. She effortlessly weaves story and sound/vibration into tools for navigating our internal wilderness. *Sacred Sound* helps us to understand and feel the archetypes that sing to us and shows us how they call us to unfold from within."

— Ana T. Forrest, creator of Forrest Yoga and author of *Fierce Medicine*

Praise for Alanna Kaivalya

"Enter yoga's secret weapon: Alanna Kaivalya.... With her knack for serving up ancient yogic philosophies in accessible ways, she is a much sought-after feature at teacher trainings around the globe. Her first book — *Myths of the Asanas*, brimming with juicy tales of love, battle, and heroism — breaks down yoga mythology and philosophy in such intriguing and accessible ways you'll never think of Dancer's Pose the same way again."

— *Sweat Equity*

Praise for *Myths of the Asanas* by Alanna Kaivalya and Arjuna van der Kooij

"Alanna and Arjuna moved down an amazing road of story and myth that truly enhances our yogic lessons. Some of the nuances of ethics, posture, breath, and meditation can only be touched through metaphor and mythology, and we thank her for taking us on this journey."

— Rodney Yee, yoga instructor and coauthor of *Yoga: The Poetry of the Body*

"What I love most about this treasure of a book is that it faithfully reminds me of the roots behind our modern-day approach to yoga. I am truly grateful to Alanna and Arjuna for providing us with such a delightfully accessible handbook on the vibrant history of our practice."

— Rusty Wells, yoga instructor and founder of Urban Flow yoga studio

"*Myths of the Asanas* transports us to a world where gods and goddesses, saints, and enlightened animals serve as our teachers. Each story reminds us that underneath the many layers of difference, essentially we are One. These inspired tales have the power to transform and revolutionize your yoga."

— MC Yogi, hip-hop artist and yoga instructor

Sacred Sound

Also by Alanna Kaivalya

Myths of the Asanas:
The Stories at the Heart of the Yoga Tradition
(with Arjuna van der Kooij)

Sacred Sound

DISCOVERING THE MYTH & MEANING OF MANTRA & KIRTAN

ALANNA KAIVALYA, PhD

FOREWORD BY DAVE STRINGER
ILLUSTRATIONS BY CHRISTOPHER YEAZEL

New World Library
Novato, California

New World Library
14 Pamaron Way
Novato, California 94949

Text design by Tona Pearce Myers
Illustrations by Christopher Yeazel

Library of Congress Cataloging-in-Publication Data
Kaivalya, Alanna, date, author.
Sacred sound : discovering the myth and meaning of mantra and kirtan / Alanna Kaivalya.
pages cm
Includes bibliographical references and index.
ISBN 978-1-60868-243-0 (paperback) — ISBN 978-1-60868-244-7 (ebook)
1. Mantras. 2. Kirtana (Hinduism) 3. Yoga. I. Title.
BL1236.36.K335 2014
294.5'37—dc23 2013046131

First printing, April 2014
ISBN 978-1-60868-243-0

Printed in Canada on 100% postconsumer-waste recycled paper

New World Library is proud to be a Gold Certified Environmentally Responsible Publisher. Publisher certification awarded by Green Press Initiative. www.greenpressinitiative.org

10 9 8 7 6 5 4 3 2

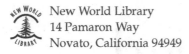

Sing in me, Muse, and through me tell the story…

— Homer

Contents

Foreword

No matter if she is teaching a workshop or holding court at a café, Alanna Kaivalya's approach to mantra, mythology, and philosophy artfully balances magic, logic, mystery, humor, and practicality. Her wide-ranging interests and her joyful unorthodoxy are among the many reasons I find her such an engaging friend and companion. So it's perfect that she conceived this book in the aftermath of an incident in which knowledge of myths and mantras turned out to be very useful.

Several years ago, Alanna, tabla player Miles Shrewsbery, and I traveled to Asia to teach and play music at a yoga training retreat. We arrived at the airport at 2 AM after a long connecting flight from Seoul. Miles and I sailed through immigration, but Alanna was not so lucky. As I was withdrawing the local currency from the cash machine in baggage claim, I was summoned by an official. Alanna had been detained. There was a problem with her passport, and they were sending her back to New York.

I was guided to a back office to discuss the situation. From the immigration officer's tone of voice, I knew right away that I was going to have to arrange some sort of "consideration" for Alanna to be admitted to the country. I'm an experienced traveler, but this was the first time I had been in this kind of situation.

My thoughts were, "How can I accomplish my aim discreetly, and not make things even more difficult than they already are?"

This part of Asia is filled with statues of the elephant-headed god Gaṇeśa (Ganesh), the lord of obstructions. To meditate on the qualities of Gaṇeśa is to observe that the way through the obstacle is often hidden in the obstacle itself. Although the immigration officer appeared to stand in our way, we understood that if we had the right attitude and paid close attention, he might also show us how to conduct ourselves. Mentally repeating the mantra *gaṇeśa śaraṇaṁ* (see the Gaṁ Gaṇapataye Namaḥ kirtan, page 159) helped us remain calm and focused.

Looking at the situation from this perspective, we could see how the officer was subtly cueing our responses every step of the way. There is no corruption in this country, he stated. So we praised his ethics, and remarked on his education. The law is strict, he said, but he himself was a compassionate man. We replied that we understood the severity of the situation, and truly regretted our ignorance of certain regulations. We acknowledged that in taking the time to find a solution to the problem with us, he had showed us consideration and respect, and we wondered if there might be a way we could show our appreciation.

Our little movie went on like this for some time. We all kept our cool and played our parts. Eventually, we were able to come to an agreement by which it was possible to receive expedited "processing." Then he disappeared for a few agonizing minutes. But he returned with a courteous smile and a freshly stamped passport, and he welcomed us to his country.

The myths and mantras of the yoga tradition are not relics gathering dust in some museum. They are flexible, practical tools that can be very helpful guides to the dilemmas of modern living. Yoga isn't a belief system; it's a method of inquiry into the nature of the mind, the heart, and the universe. It's also an oral tradition that emphasizes practice and experience. The mantras are meant to be sung and spoken until the practitioner becomes their very embodiment. You start out chanting the mantras, but after a while, they start to chant you.

You can read all the books you want about swimming, but you won't really learn anything about it until you dive into the water. Repeat these mantras, and see what they bring up for you. Observe what kind of changes you experience in your perceptions and your reactions. The elemental sounds of these mantras can stimulate a subtle range of feeling states, and the stories can open windows with a view to elemental truths.

Story is our essence, the source and expression of every vision, fear, dream, death, birth, and discovery. Our humanity and inhumanity are rooted in it, embedded in the mystery of "why?" and the suspense of "what next?" Story is nature's way of becoming conscious of itself, and it's the way we build our consciousness, too.

We still lack a complete definition and understanding of what consciousness is, but we can say that there is no direct, objective experience of reality. Confronting a mass of neural blips, buzzing energy, and sensory perceptions, the brain finds patterns, sorts things into categories, and searches for meaning. It creates stories, and in making stories, it makes the world tangible and real to us.

In this accessible guide, Alanna shows some of the ways that myths and mantras can enrich our inner lives, and gives us an informed approach to meaningful living. I'm pleased to have been in her circle when the ideas for this book were germinating, and proud that she has produced such a lucid and entertaining manuscript. I hope that everyone who reads this book will be able to see the mantras reflected in themselves and see their own lives as vehicles of meaning and joy. These mantras are the essential stories of us all.

Dave Stringer,
kirtan singer and performing artist

Introduction

Many years ago when I started a yoga practice, I had no idea what it would reveal to me. I was just hoping for a little extra strength and flexibility, and I did what I could to avoid all the spiritual trappings of the practice. But, somehow, as it does, the yoga did its job. Over the years it brought me through physical, psychological, and emotional revelations that I can't imagine would have taken place otherwise.

One of the most powerful insights has come through the use of sound and mantra as a basis for the practice. I was born with a hearing impairment that gave me a unique relationship to sound. As a child, I would feel sound, vibration, tone, and intonation in order to more fully access my world. This was second nature to me, but through my studies of yoga (and physics!), I suddenly found a reason behind my special relationship to sound. Just as important, through yoga's rich mythology, I also gained context and meaning to better understand how the inner and outer practices of yoga work. It is from this perspective that I have always practiced and taught, fueled by the belief that sound has the power to harmonize us and myth brings forth what is alive within us. It is in this spirit that I always end my lectures and workshops with these words: Don't miss the vibrations.

This book covers a lot of ground. It presents twenty-one mantras or chants that stem from our yogic tradition — some with tremendous historicity and some that are more modern derivations. It also describes the myth, text, or context each mantra comes from or is associated with, and it explains how these rich myths relate to our modern-day spiritual practice.

My hope is that, with this guide, you will come to use these chants in your spiritual practice in a variety of ways. In your personal practice, you may chant in order to fuel your meditation, with or without accompaniment (sometimes chanting to yourself in the shower is as uplifting as chanting on the floor with a harmonium!). If you are a yoga student, you may discover that these chants come up in your classes or in the music the instructor plays. If you are a teacher, these chants can be used as jumping-off points for enriching classroom discussions of yogic wisdom and lively mythology. Even if your yoga practice includes zero *āsana* (physical postures), you can use these chants as your sole spiritual practice. Let their vibrations and related myths uplift your mind, outlook, and sense of well-being to generate an overall feeling of harmony. There is no wrong way to utilize these chants and bring them into your own spiritual practice. Let them help and support you on your spiritual journey.

The mantras, their corresponding myths, and the spiritual guidance they contain are all connected through vibration, which is encompassed through the practice of *nāda* yoga. The principle of *nāda* yoga — the yoga of sacred sound — plays a key role in any type of yoga practice and is held sacred in all yoga practices. In yoga, making a personal connection with the source is paramount, and it is held that the nature of the source is vibration. Wherever we look in yoga practice, we find the reference to this internal, sacred sound, known as *nāda*. The *nāda* is said to arise from the heart and is the vibrational equivalent of our own personal *oṁ* (ॐ). In order to access this sound, and refine our internal listening to connect with it, we start by refining and tuning up our outer listening. This can include both the acts of listening to music as well as making music. The yogi enhances this dynamic interaction with sound through mantra. Mantras work on not only the mind and attitude of the chanter (or listener!) but on the internal energetic body of the chanter (and listener). As we harmonize our mind and body through the chants and bring into tune our psyche and heart through the mythology, we create a self that is in sync with our highest vibration.

In this book, by weaving together chants, tales, and spiritual philosophy, I hope to give you a feeling-sense of how the vibrations are brought to life by the mantra, how the mantra is vivified by the story, and how we are enlivened through the embodiment of the myth and mantra. This isn't merely a theory to understand but a practice meant to be fully embodied and experienced. The transformative power of vibration is something you must feel and verify for yourself. There is no wisdom that is more important than the self-evident wisdom that arises when we put theory into practice.

Mantras and Chants

A mantra, as it relates to the yogic and Vedic traditions of India, is a Sanskrit phrase that encapsulates some higher idea or ideal within the cadence, vibration, and essence of its sound. A mantra can be as simple as a single sound — such as chanting the well-known sound *oṁ* — or as complicated as chanting a poem that tells a grand story or gives instruction. Whatever mantra is chanted, no matter how long or short, the purpose is the same: it is meant to act like a skeleton key to help you bypass the mundane matters and mental chatter of the day-to-day mind in order to reach a transcendent state of awareness and self-realization that is, quite frankly, indescribable. Every yogic practice provides the means for us to do this — such as *āsana* (postures), meditation, and *prāṇāyāma* (breath work) — but mantra practice and *nāda* yoga are uniquely simple and universal. If you can form a thought, you can do a mantra practice. The simple act of *thinking* a mantra is a start to a genuine practice. The silent repetition of the sound *oṁ* while driving, for example, can be a starting point. Eventually, our practice might grow to include chanting while meditating, attending lively mantra-based musical performances (kirtan, or *kīrtana*), or perhaps even chanting a longer mantra 108 times aloud to celebrate the New Year. As I've said, there is no wrong way to use a mantra.

In the United States, mantra has gained popularity largely through the musical kirtan (*kīrtana*) tradition. Popular kirtan musicians such as Krishna Das, Deva Premal, and Dave Stringer have brought these Eastern chants to life by giving them some good old American rock-and-roll flair. While the kirtan tradition in India began around the ninth century, its look and feel hasn't changed much even as it has evolved to incorporate Western musical proclivities. It has always had (and still has) a fairly simplistic call-and-response-type format, where the leader will chant a phrase that is repeated by the audience. This typically becomes more lively and fast as the chant continues. In India, various instruments are used — typically the harmonium (similar to an accordion in a box), the tabla (classical Indian drum set), and the cartals (tiny cymbals). Those instruments are still present in many kirtan settings today, yet the music is often Westernized through the incorporation of all sorts of instruments, like the guitar, bass, and even a proper Western drum kit (like how Chris Grosso and I perform!). What is wonderful about many of these yogic and Vedic traditions is that they are quite malleable. So long as the intention is still sealed within the practice, the practice — even if it is modernized and Westernized — does not lose its efficacy.

So while some choose to chant mantras in a kirtan setting, others have long used mantra in spiritual practice in accordance with daily rituals, meditation, or as a way to bind fellow students of a tradition. Many use a mantra during their morning worship practice to invoke an intention or particular deity. Many practitioners also stay focused in their meditation practice by silently or quietly chanting a mantra. And some traditions claim certain mantras as part of their tradition — almost like a secret handshake. In many Eastern spiritual traditions, it is common at the beginning and end of a spiritual practice to chant a mantra or *oṁ*. Mantras are also commonly used as prayers for peace, health, or well-being. Mantras can be used to focus the mind and empower whatever spiritual practice we embark on. Mantra is fuel for the inner spiritual fire.

In truth, you don't need to know or do anything more to use mantras in your own daily practice, but don't be afraid to experiment and try something new. Read through all the mantras in this book. Say them out loud. If any resonate with you, keep using them. Sometimes people are reluctant to chant mantras they don't know the meaning of, but that is one reason I wrote this book! Also, keep in mind that there are many more mantras than appear in this book, and all are efficacious. Mantras are beneficial compilations of vibration that help to uplift you.

Finally, if you are brand-new to yoga or Eastern spiritual practices, know that chanting mantras doesn't make you a Hindu. By chanting, you are not joining a religion or expressing your belief in any religious dogma. The aim is spiritual, not denominational. The power of mantra lies in the vibrations, and these vibrations work on many levels, whether the sayings are pronounced out loud or silently, correctly or incorrectly. The benefits of chanting do increase with more accurate pronunciation — just as pronouncing any foreign language correctly makes it more intelligible — as well as with better understanding of the meanings, but the simple act of saying a mantra will still bring the mind and heart into alignment with its subtle goal, which is to bring heightened self-awareness and a deeper sense of peace and calm.

With that in mind, I encourage you to simply begin a mantra practice in whatever way that feels right, using this book as a guide. Start simple, such as with *oṁ*, and incorporate other, longer, or more complex mantras as they resonate with you. Some mantras may appeal to you because of their sound, while others may become attractive as you understand their context, underlying mythology, and intention. Over time, as you use each mantra in your life and practice, it will become like a friend whom you come to know more and more deeply. The mantra may start out as a little gem that lightens your day, but after years of saying it, it may also become a bright light that guides you through the darkest of times. Through practice, we make these mantras our own so they help us on our spiritual journey.

The Historical Context of Mantra Practice

The mantras compiled in this book come from a variety of sources within the vast scope of the Vedic tradition. The Vedic tradition is a broad term that defines the text and rituals coming out of the historic Indus Valley, and it is based on one of the world's most ancient spiritual texts: the Veda (a.k.a. Vedas). Many Vedic texts are said to have been simply "received" by ancient saints (called *rishis* or *ṛṣi*) as opposed to being authored by a specific person. It is from the tradition of the Veda that we derive the original practice of mantra. These historic source texts were founts of wisdom that were unlocked by those who could read them — namely the Vedic priests. They would bring the knowledge and tradition of the texts to the people via ritual chanting and fire ceremonies. Even today, chants like the Gāyatrī Mantra (page 65) are largely unchanged from their Vedic roots.

Over time, other important source texts arose within the Eastern spiritual traditions, and more mantras emerged from them. For example, the Purāṇa (Puranas) are the source of much of the mythic history of the East. They contain mantras and have been the source of inspiration for modern mantras. Many of our current spiritual and yogic leaders in the West have looked to the Purāṇa for mythic inspiration, and they have written simple kirtan chants to invoke the energy and essence of various iconic deities. Mantras also embody the focus of specific spiritual traditions. For example, the Mahā Mantra (page 153) of the Krishna Consciousness tradition helps practitioners enliven and enlighten their spiritual quest for a deep, internal relationship with Krishna (Kṛṣṇa).

Mantra represents an unbelievably accessible and widespread tradition, one that extends from the millennia-old mantras of the Veda, which are chanted widely in yoga class and teacher trainings, to the contemporary composers of the kirtan tradition, who have brought mantra to life with a Western twist. Mantras remain popular in today's spiritual practices, and yet modern-day spiritual practitioners have had no single resource that brought them together and illuminated them. I hope this book fills that need, for after all, knowledge is power. Tracing these venerable vibrations to their source shows us not only the history of the yogic practice but also how we have evolved it and moved it forward to suit our current needs and cultural matrix. Because mantras are of no use if they don't speak to our modern-day psyche.

Mantra Categories and the Yogic Tradition

The mantras in this book are divided into two sections, which I have labeled "Classic Mantras" and "Traditional Kirtan." These categories are loose and unofficial, but they help distinguish two basic types of mantra. The classic mantras tend to come from older Vedic or yogic source texts, and they tend to be chanted during yoga practice without musical accompaniment. The traditional kirtans are almost always deity-focused chants that are often used within the lively, musical kirtan tradition, and they incorporate call-and-response chanting. Kirtans may have no specific textual derivation and may even be rather recently derived. In any case, these mantra categories are not absolute. You may find that one mantra could easily fit within the other category, for as you may have gathered by now, there are few rules within this tradition and many exceptions. The labels are not important, for there isn't just one correct way to chant a mantra. As I say, you can adapt them freely in whatever way enhances your own practice.

Each mantra entry also introduces the source text for the chant (if it has one) and suggests how to interpret or think of the chant's meaning. When discussing source texts, I commonly refer to the "yogic" and "Vedic" traditions, but for this book, they are largely one and the same. The Veda is the source of all yogic traditions, and I am interpreting the mantras from a yogic point of view. Simply put, a yogic point of view looks at the esoteric or mystical meaning. Nowhere in this book will any of these texts be referenced as religious doctrine. Rather, I explore the mantras — and the source texts they come from — as sources of inward-turning inspiration. That is the yogic aim, and it is maintained throughout.

A Word about Sanskrit, Translations, and Spellings

Vedic and yogic mantras are all based in the language of Sanskrit (Saṁskṛta). In this book, I include three versions of every chant: the proper Sanskrit, a transliterated version (which is the version you speak), and the English translation. However, I have also taken care to use the transliterated spellings for most of the important and commonly used Sanskrit words, and I have included a select glossary at the end of the book. Sometimes, to ease understanding, I've put the English spelling in parenthesis after transliterated Sanskrit. However, a few Sanskrit words are now so widely adopted within the English language that I have left them unitalicized, even though they are spelled the same in transliterated Sanskrit, such as yoga, mantra, karma, dharma, bhakti, and guru.

Interestingly, when writing this book, deciding when to follow accepted English usage and when to maintain proper Sanskrit proved a challenge. For example, properly transliterated Sanskrit words are generally not capitalized or pluralized, but that bucks with the sensibilities of English grammar. While I have usually used Sanskrit spellings and diacritics, I've deferred to American styling of proper names, so that they appear roman and capitalized. I think this simply makes for easier reading. What I hope is that the approach in this book strikes a happy medium between readability and faithfulness to the original source language of the yoga tradition.

The reason for including the transliterated Sanskrit is simple: this book is about sacred sound. In this tradition, sacred sound is fueled by the language of Sanskrit, which is a vibrational language that expresses the essence of what it describes. For example, the Sanskrit word *abhaya* is often translated as "fearlessness." But the word is not merely that. It is the state of being fearless as well as the fortified attitude with which one has strived to achieve this state, and the way one is received when this state is embodied. *Abhaya* expresses all of these things effortlessly through the vibration of the word itself, which if repeated over and over (like a mantra) will eventually communicate its essential meaning within us. We will *feel* the word's power start to shift us so that we embody the state of fearlessness. Understanding this essential, vibrational power of Sanskrit lends potency to our practice of mantra and chanting.

There is great magic in the source language of yoga. In his book *The Power of Myth*, scholar Joseph Campbell describes Sanskrit as "the great spiritual language of the world." Indeed, all of yoga's primary texts are written in Sanskrit, and there is great benefit in stretching one's mind to incorporate what the original vibrations contained. Otherwise, things can become lost in translation. Just like dating someone whose native tongue is not your own, learning this foreign language will give greater understanding and strengthen the shared bond between you and yoga.

As for the mantras, even with the Sanskrit transliterations, they can appear like tongue twisters. So much of mantra practice is about pronunciation, so it may take some time and dedicated practice to develop a true comfort level during chanting. To this end, audio files of every mantra in this book (plus more!) are available online on my website at http://alannak.com/musicians-mantras/mantra-library. These sacred mantras have great value in and of themselves as conductors of sacred vibration, but they also have philosophical value in what they impart to the yoga practitioner. While all of the mantras (from both sections) contain a variety of the forty-nine unique sounds in the

Sanskrit language, their messages contain unique and specific information for the chanter. Whether we derive this information through the vibrations of the chant itself, through understanding the meaning of the words, or by embodying what the mantra puts forth, these mantras are containers of yogic wisdom that enhance not only our practice but who we are as human beings.

How to Chant: Some Practical Instructions

As I've said, there are no hard and fast rules for chanting. It can be done silently or aloud, in a group or on one's own. The act of speaking the mantra (even silently) allows the mantra to do its job. However, you can strengthen and improve your practice by also focusing on the meaning of the mantra and pronouncing the Sanskrit correctly. Even so, without any intention and with halting pronunciation, you will still derive a benefit from a mantra practice, just as for someone trying to get into shape, any exercise is good exercise.

Whether you are new to chanting or not, here are some general tips for chanting and for developing or improving your mantra practice:

To start, practice one chant consistently for as little as five minutes a day. It could be a vocalized repetition of the sound of *oṁ* in the shower, or quietly repeating the Gāyatrī Mantra upon waking. Get into the habit of speaking Sanskrit regularly. Get used to the patterns and sounds, and soon the chants will come more easily and naturally. Match saying the mantra with the regular, steady rhythm of your breath. This will help the mantra to regulate your autonomic functions and put your breath, body, and mind into better alignment. If you practice this regularly, you may find that the mantra appears in your head throughout the day as a touchstone of steadiness and stillness. That's great — it means the mantra is working!

Choose a chant that resonates with you, and incorporate it within a meditation practice. If you don't already have a meditation practice, starting one is actually very simple. Find a quiet, comfortable place, sit up nice and tall, and close your eyes. Then either silently or quietly chant the mantra. If you haven't memorized the chant, lay this book out in front of you, open to the proper page, and say the mantra over and over until there is a natural flow. While you chant, let the mantra fall into rhythm with the pattern of your breath. If you are saying the mantra out loud, focus on the vowels, as this is the source of the most powerful resonance. If it helps, place one hand over your heart to feel the vibrations inside your chest.

While there is no wrong way to chant a mantra, it is nice to adopt a style or mode that is either "common" or "traditional." The style of Vedic chanting has only three tones: the one you speak at, one tone above, and one tone below. This makes it easy for everyone — no matter what your voice sounds like — to try and chant. A good example is the Asato Mā chant, which you can find online in my website's mantra library (http://alannak.com/musicians-mantras/mantra-library). It is a prime example of this style of Vedic chanting. Some modern-day teachers and kirtan singers make the mantras sound fancy and more singsongy, but they don't need to be. Start simple. Find a rhythm and a tone that works for you and keep at it.

If you like kirtan — the lively practice of call-and-response chanting set to uplifting music — sing along! Seriously. Put on a kirtan CD and sing along as if you are part of the crowd. The great music of the kirtan style will liven up your mantra practice, and if the spirit moves you, grab a tambourine, stomp your feet, clap your hands, and let the spirit of the mantra carry you away. Chanting kirtan is typically call-and-response, but this doesn't mean you can't do both the call and the response. If you're alone, sing all the parts to yourself. When kirtan chanting is done in groups (such as in yoga class or at a concert), a leader "calls" and the audience "responds." It is a simple practice — it is meant to be. This helps make it universal and accessible.

If you attend a yoga class, kirtan, or *satsaṅga* (a.k.a. satsang, a spiritually-based group event), you may find that the teacher will chant a mantra differently than you learned it. If so, just go with the flow and focus on the vibration and intention of the chant. You may even discover that you like this version better! Also, some mantra practitioners believe that there is only one correct way to chant each mantra, but this just isn't so. If this were the case, then mantras would only be efficacious when chanted in a particular way, and there is no evidence for this. The most traditional Vedic schools of chanting maintain a simple rhythm and pattern for some mantras, but those mantras can also be dressed up in a kirtan-type setting. Not only is this okay and appropriate, but it can breathe new life into them!

Whether chanted in a traditional or modern setting, on your own or in yoga class, with or without music, silently or aloud, mantra will move you. It will touch the deepest parts of yourself that few other spiritual disciplines can reach. Start with a mantra practice that feels comfortable and expand your horizons from there.

Same Source, Separate Traditions: Yoga and Hinduism

The universality of these mantras might be one of the reasons why they (and their source texts) have stood the test of time. While many spiritual traditions have songs or chants that express wholeness, compassion, and unity, the eloquence with which Vedic and yogic mantras express these uplifted human values has a lyrical quality that unlocks the heart of the practitioner in ways that we cannot imagine, but only experience. While the mantras have long been practiced as a part of the yogic tradition, the growing popularity of yoga in the West has made them accessible as exceptional tools to heighten the experience of our spiritual practice. As the mystical arm of the larger Vedic tradition, yoga is a way to enhance our spiritual depth and strengthen our belief system, even if it differs from yoga's Vedic origins.

Yoga evolved around the Vedic and Hindu cultures in India, and so its wisdom incorporates a lot of the same language, mythology, and philosophy. However, yoga differs in that it points the practitioner inward, to the mystical or esoteric source of internal spirituality, similar to the way that Gnosticism does within the Christian tradition, Sufism within the Islamic tradition, and Kabbalah within the Jewish tradition. While certainly related to Hinduism, yoga doesn't require participants to embody the religious aspects of the Hindu tradition. This is similar to the way people — like Madonna! — have incorporated Kabbalistic practices into their daily repertoire in order to enhance their spiritual well-being. In general, the mystical traditions of most religions are designed to lead us inward, to our highest state of being, rather than outward to an externalized expression of faith.

Though yoga evolved alongside Hinduism and is sourced from the same Vedic wisdom, their intentions are fundamentally different. Yoga leads practitioners to an internalized, mystical, and esoteric understanding of their highest self. Hinduism focuses outward to the more traditional and canonical structure of the faith. Like a pair of siblings who grew up in the same household, one an extrovert and one an introvert, Hinduism and yoga have a shared history and a common goal, but different means of getting their points and practices across. So, while many of the myths, texts, and philosophical underpinnings found in this book may have a shared relevance across the Vedic, yogic, and Hindu traditions, our point of view will be through the yogic lens — the lens that shows the internal structure of our highest self.

The Universality of Yogic Mythology

One of the exceptional aspects of the yoga tradition is its all-inclusive nature. It accepts all practitioners, no matter what their original spiritual or religious background, and helps them experience the numinous in their lives. But, because the numinous cannot be named or described, the number one way in which this kind of psychological and spiritual information is conveyed is through mythology.

Mythology is the language of the unconscious. It gives shape, meaning, and context to the archetypes of the collective unconscious, and that allows us, in turn, to give shape, meaning, and context to the stories that play out within our lives. Mythology is an essential part of our human psyche. And it is critical to cultivate a meaningful mythology within each of our lives. This is particularly important in our modern world, when so few traditions, religious and otherwise, provide this. Perhaps we grew up within a religious tradition that, for whatever reason, we have since walked away from, but it is important that we still continue journeying *toward* a mythology that enlivens our psyche — that gives our life meaning. We need to find out, as Carl Jung asked himself, what myth we are living by.

What is a myth? Put most simply, myth is metaphor. Joseph Campbell often described myth this way. As he explained, through metaphor, we are better able to understand ourselves and the world. For example, in the myth of the Bhagavad Gītā, the hero Arjuna has an intense dialogue with his chariot driver, Kṛṣṇa (Krishna). Arjuna is about to go into battle, and seeing that his enemy's army is both enormous and partly composed of his family and friends, he is filled with doubt and tries to chicken out (for more on this story, see the Mahā Mantra, page 153). This metaphor speaks to all of us. We can all imagine ourselves as Arjuna, faced with the challenge of the spiritual journey. As we cope with our own fears and doubts as we approach our life's battles, we can turn to the myth of Arjuna to provide a meaningful perspective on our own situation. Myths aren't necessarily true in the empirical sense — even when they refer to real, historical figures and actual events. Myths embody deeper truths about the nature of life, and they often embody important guidance or life lessons. Myths bring meaning to our lives and help us to navigate life's difficulties like an old friend leading us by the hand. From the yogic perspective, myths help guide us on the journey inward, which is possibly the most fruitful journey there is.

Mythology helps us cultivate and deepen the relationship between the ego and the higher self, between ourselves and those we love, and it helps us bring forth what is alive within us into the world. Mythology gives us the tools, means, characters, rites, context, and lessons so that we can then live, embody, vivify, and restore the verve to our life.

As it turns out, the yogic tradition has awesome mythology. The rich stories found within the original source texts — whose history spans millennia and whose true authors remain cloaked in mystery — help shed light on the challenges, trials, and tribulations of life. While precise dates are largely unknown, we surmise that the Vedas, widely regarded as the world's oldest known spiritual texts, are at least five thousand years old. The Vedas laid the extensive groundwork for the Indus Valley tradition, but beginning somewhere around 1500 BCE, their grand scope was eventually distilled into the more concise spiritual texts known as the Upaniṣad (Upanishads). Around the start of the Common Era, we start to find the riches of the story-filled Purāṇa (Puranas). All of these texts feature an enormous body of rich mythology that provides us with fantastic metaphors for life and the human condition.

Though these truths are universal, the shapes that they take within the yogic mythological tradition are highly varied. There are said to be 300 million gods in the Vedic pantheon. Alain Daniélou, author of *The Myths and the Gods of India: The Classic Work on Hindu Polytheism*, states it eloquently this way:

> Hindu mythology acknowledges all gods. Since all the energies at the origin of all the forms of manifestation are but aspects of the divine power, there can exist no object, no form of existence, which is not divine in nature. Any name, any shape, that appeals to the worshipper can be taken as a representation or manifestation of divinity.

In other words, all manifestations of yogic mythology are simply reflections of one numinous source, and they provide endless avenues by which we can discover that source within ourselves. Or, as Eknath Easwaran, student of Gandhi and founder of the Blue Mountain Center of Meditation, once described this, "Yogic myth has the genius to cloak the infinite in human form."

Archetypes, Mythology, and the Unconscious

The infinite is indeed within. Deep in our own psyche — within everyone's psyche — lives the framework of the human journey. These structural archetypes are the substructure of thousands of years of our collective hopes, dreams, desires, failures, and fears. These archetypal, shared experiences of the collective unconscious provide a common architecture for the stories — that is, the myths — we tell ourselves about our humanity, about our struggles and triumphs. When dressed up, brought to life, and vivified through our imagination, our mythic stories allow us to witness what is deeply inside us at play in front of us. Myths give us the context and the capability to bring our inner world *out*. This is actually a critical part of our psycho-spiritual development process. As we delve into our spiritual practice, what we discover within will need to come up and out. The spiritual journey of the yoga practitioner will bring us face-to-face with the inner reaches of our unconscious — the part of our mind that is not known to us, which includes not just the autonomic functions, but the hidden drives behind nearly every action and reaction. Once we go inward, myths help us to bear everything we discover by giving our internal elements context. We gain a greater understanding of their nature and place in our lives.

What exactly are the things in our unconscious that myths help us see? Basically, anything (and all the things) we don't want to look at about ourselves. These might be positive aspects of ourselves that we don't want to admit, but most often these are the negative aspects that we refuse to acknowledge. This is our dark side, what Carl Jung would call our "shadow," made up of the things that we have repressed, ignored, or otherwise left in the unconscious to be discovered at a later time. The question, though, when that later time arises, is will we be ready and willing to look at that shadow? And will we invite that shadow to come forth and show us where we are still not free? As long as what is buried in the unconscious remains there, it will prevent us from unleashing our full potential.

Spiritual transformation, particularly in Eastern spiritual practices, asks us to *delve into the dark side*. Nobody likes it. It's not popular. But every hero in every mythic tradition has to uncover and explore their own dark side in order to discover their light. Many people in spiritual traditions today tend to be so focused on their light that they leave no room for the potent power of the shadow to show them what is really alive within them. Think about Luke Skywalker when he is being trained by Yoda on Dagobah in *The Empire Strikes Back*. Yoda tells Luke to enter a cave, where he must slay his greatest fear. First, Darth Vader appears, but after Luke beheads the Sith lord, the mask cracks open to reveal Luke's own face inside. The true nature of what Luke fears the most is not Darth Vader but rather his own darkness, fear, and anger. Overcoming this personal darkness is the hero's greatest task, and it's important because, as Carl Jung is rumored to have said, "until you make the unconscious conscious, it will direct your life and you will call it fate." Until we bring forth what is lying in the unconscious, we are ignoring the part of ourselves that brings this world to life.[1]

Mythology does that for us. It accesses the parts of our psyche that are yearning for a voice and expression. Through myth, we can come to know all the parts of our self and learn to accept ourselves entirely — the good, the bad, and the ugly. In our spiritual journey, mythology gives us the footing we need to navigate the rocky crags and sketchy footholds of what lies inside of us. As we delve inward, we discover that these seemingly dangerous territories are actually the tempered structures that give us a formidable strength that allows us to navigate anything. Through myths, we see that what was once a dangerous cliff is an opportunity to soar, and what was once a great monster is our greatest ally.

Further, while mythic archetypes are by definition enduring, their meanings are not scripted. They can have different meanings for different people. In this way, the metaphorical power of myth is both universal and specific; it places each of us within the context of the larger human journey and also helps us make sense of our individual, personal, and unique journey. Myths are neither factual reports nor dogmatic, rigid lessons that can only be interpreted and understood in one way.

How this works is a mystery, and author Joachim-Ernst Berendt, in his book *The World Is Sound: Nada Brahma,* captures this well when he writes, "To our western mind, legends and myths hail from ancient times, but the only reason they do so is because we have banished them there. In reality, they are *now.* They have come into existence because people need them. The rationalist believes he can do without myths. He doesn't want to be made uncertain of his 'belief' that the rational mind is omnipotent."

We need mythology, and we need what mythology brings to us: hope, inspiration, and meaning. We can find this when we embrace the truth of myth without needing it to be factually true. Literalizing myth removes its inherent universality, and it is precisely this mysterious quality of enduring malleability that enlivens myth and enables it to be meaningful for us.

The Music of the Spheres

Through the mantras and myths in this book, you will discover a vibrancy and illumination that will enliven your life and outlook. All the elements of the practice — the sounds of the words themselves, the vocalized chanting, and the mythic understandings the mantras represent — elevate consciousness and are cohesively bound together with the power of vibration. One of the great links between the conscious and unconscious — and between human beings, cultures, and even particles in our universe — is the power of vibration and sound. This is the core thread that holds our experience and understanding together. It's uncanny how everything is cradled in vibration — whether lying in wait to be born as something new, brought to life by the music of the spheres, or transformed forever by the unifying power of harmony. Throughout time and across the world (and the universe), we are bound together by music. Through chanting and sacred sound, we discover a force that unifies us that is both explainable, measurable, and numinous in its affective quality and inspiration. In fact, as Candace Alcorta writes, "the human ability to make and be moved by music is a universal human trait. Like miracles, music is intimately interconnected with a sense of the sacred, the numinous, and the divine. Music not only represents the sacred; it also calls it forth and embodies it, as well."[2]

Music has the unique power to unite. If we learn to harness the power of music and its underlying vibration, we can use it to elevate our own state of awareness as well as to develop our interconnectedness with the world around us. Music is hardwired into our brain. Despite the fact that, evolutionarily speaking, humans have no need for music, as Alcorta writes, "humans are born with the genetically encoded neural structures necessary for the analysis and processing of the acoustic, pitch, and temporal properties of music." So music is not a frivolous aspect of our humanity, but rather an innate part of who we are. All of us have the ability to recognize, listen to, and enjoy music. Through music and sound, we elevate our mood, connect with others, and enliven our spirits. In a room full of music, something magical happens. It's called *entrainment*.

This is such a fantastic word.

Entrainment is the process of vibrations falling into sync with one another, which happens because the universe tends toward harmony. The technical term is "mutual phase-locking" and its ramifications for us are significant. When two oscillators are pulsating in the same field, they "lock in" to the same rhythm and become entrained. If two muscle cells from a human heart are placed next to each other in a petri dish, they will eventually pulsate in the same rhythm — and two people sitting close together will also discover their heartbeats (and breath!) eventually coincide. A good lecturer with a captivated audience will cause the brain wave function of the audience to lock into phase together. Entrainment also describes how large schools of fish move in tandem with one another, never colliding, as do flocks of birds.

As Joachim-Ernst Berendt writes, it seems that "entering into harmonic relationships is the goal not only of music, it is the goal of atoms and molecules, of planetary orbits, of cells and hearts, of brain waves and movements, of flocks of birds and schools of fish and — in principle — of human beings. All of them (or better: the cosmos, the entire creation) have harmony as their final goal. They are all moving to realize Nāda Brahmā, the world is sound."[3]

It's no wonder that mantra, kirtan, and the music we make with our own heartbeats is powerful medicine to heal the schism of the psyche and the split of disconnection that is the source of much disease. The sacred vibrations and sounds of the Sanskrit language, in particular, are an anecdote for the anomalous vibrations that give rise to discord and a feeling of being "out of sync" with our thoughts, words, and actions. These sacred sounds empower us to realize the harmony that is quite literally *waiting* to be recalibrated within us and to reconnect with the symphony of hearts that occupy a room of people chanting together. No wonder we feel better after chanting *oṁ* (ॐ), or participating in a kirtan, or meditating with a mantra. Sacred sound and vibration access the fundamental pulsation of our life energy and bring it into accord with the entirety of our being.

This is how the yoga always does its job.

It realigns our spirit. It calls forth that which is alive inside of us. It reintegrates the lost parts of our psyche and vivifies our hopes and dreams while synthesizing all that we've tried to block out, helping us to recognize that everything is awesomely okay.

Mythology takes us into the depths of our inner self, reveals hidden truths, and then leads us back out again. Sacred sound reintegrates all the parts of the self so that we can find balance and harmony both within and without. By discovering the mythology *behind* the mantras, we have the complete means to discover the most fundamental teaching of yoga — that we are whole, complete, and perfect just as we are.

In this spirit, I bring these wonderful myths and mantras to you.

Don't miss the vibrations.

PART ONE

Classic Mantras

The mantra tradition is extremely old. In fact, the oldest mantras are said to predate any recorded history and to have come to us through the ages, having been passed down from teacher to student since time immemorial. One mantra, *oṁ*, is even said to have been present before time began — for *oṁ* was the catalyst that shaped the universe.

Throughout history, mantras have been crafted to illuminate what is alive within us: our vast human potential that needs only the right key to be unlocked. These ancient mantras are said to be that key. Whether ancient or merely very old, the power of these mantras lies in their vibrational structure and hidden meaning.

The so-called classic mantras in this part have come to us from the wide variety of source texts that make up the yogic and Vedic traditions. Their history has given them time to percolate and gain strength over the long years as people have chanted them to catalyze their spiritual practice. This kind of power, focused through the vibration of the chant itself, is a way to supercharge our practice and "plug in" to the source of yoga in the same way we recharge our iPods at night. When we chant these mantras, it is like we are accessing a current of sound. It is a river whose waters will carry us through the transformational aspects of a spiritual practice.

As I've said, the designation "classic mantras" is my own, and I've used it to distinguish the popular mantras that have a strong presence in our Western yoga tradition from the mantras in part two that are typically chanted in kirtan. The mantras in this section are not specific to a certain time or text, but they tend to be older (some are said to be timeless, like the Gāyatrī Mantra), and they are more intricate than the more simplistic kirtan chants. However, you might hear some of these mantras in a kirtan setting, too. Most of these classic mantras are generally used for meditation, *satsaṅga*, or personal practice outside of a musical setting. Some are also strongholds of specific traditions, such as the mantras of initiation used to include a practitioner within the folds of a spiritual group. That said, these mantras are not exclusive to one tradition, either. They are sometimes found in multiple texts and have been widely adored by yoga practitioners for as long as they've been in circulation.

These chants often address or focus on the teachers, students, lovers, and beloveds of the yoga tradition. Some chants are explicit in their inherent meaning, and some chants are more like Zen koans — they need time and the powers of a quiet mind to crack. But all of these chants have a powerful history and derive from powerful sources. These chants come from the Veda (Vedas), the Upaniṣad (Upanishads), the Purāṇa (Puranas), and even some more specific yogic texts like the Yoga Taravāli. These sources — each in their own way — help to illuminate the basic configuration of the Vedic tradition, and the specific mantras are highlights of those sources. They are focused phrases that reveal powerful human truths. They tend to be a bit more structured, and their meanings come to us largely from the source text we find them in. These mantras mean business, and as such, they act as vibrational guideposts in our spiritual practice.

In a way, these classic mantras are like challenging teachers who set a high bar. But eventually they will become like old friends who remind us of who we are and what we might still be hiding or holding on to. This process takes time. Embarking on a mantra practice is like starting an exercise program. It may be difficult at first — trying out new pronunciations or words, finding time to incorporate the chants into your practice. Yet eventually, these sacred vibrations will work their magic, recalibrating our internal system so that their teachings are not just intellectually understood but *known* and *felt* within our body and our spirit. Over time, they will take up residence in our heart, so that we emanate their profound teachings from within every time we step off our mat or rise from our cushion. Eventually, we stop chanting the mantra, and the mantra starts chanting us.

Get to know these mantras. Hang out with them for a while. They are worthwhile teachers on this spiritual path. They are great aides in guiding us home.

1. Oṁ

The most basic, fundamental mantra is the sound *oṁ* (ॐ). We are not sure when the sound *oṁ* first made its appearance in the minds of the ancient sages and was written down in the Veda, but it is thought to have been present at the beginning of the universe. Within it, we find the source vibrations of the entire Sanskrit language, kind of like the "alpha and the omega." Chanting *oṁ* helps us to realign ourselves with the fundamental vibration present within all things and sets the stage for harmony.

ॐ
oṁ

Advice for Chanting

Oṁ is the sacred sound of the universe. It can literally be chanted anywhere, anytime, out loud or silently. It is highly effective in bringing into harmony a space, your body, an idea, or your spiritual practice. Often, it is chanted to start and end a practice, but it could also be used in other creative settings. *Oṁ* could be chanted before a meal to harmonize everyone at the table, in the middle of writer's block to clear your head and allow creativity to flow, or in any situation that needs a little more centering, peace, and calm. It will impart balance in any way to match your intention.

In order to make the sound of *oṁ*, round the lips into an O shape and drop the jaw a bit. Let the tongue relax and clear lots of space in the mouth and throat as the sound is made. Pronounce *oṁ* as in "home," as opposed to "aum" as in "prom" — despite the explanation of *oṁ* that follows. This is because, in Sanskrit, both the sounds of A and U are incorporated into the O sound, so all the metaphorical bases are covered.

When chanting, spend the first part of the extended exhale on the O sound. Feel its resonance in your face and head, and even place a hand on the chest to feel the resonance inside the heart. About halfway through the breath, close the lips and make the M sound. Experience the vibrations as they rise to the crown of the head. The vibrational nature of *oṁ* brings the current of sound up from the depths of your being all the way through your physical form and out the crown of the head. This is a complete experience of the powerful vibration of sacred sound and is at the heart of the yoga tradition.

Oṁ Is Where the Heart Is

At the heart of the yoga tradition lies the fundamental teaching that within us all we are an interconnected web with no broken threads, as in the mythical net of Indra, which is cast over the entire universe and has a gem at each juncture. If that web were to vibrate, we would feel it in our heart, and it would resonate with the sound of *oṁ* (ॐ).

Oṁ is made up of four sounds: A, U, M, and silence. In Sanskrit, the complex vowel O is made when the sounds A and U combine to make the full and complete sound of O. So, the first two parts of *oṁ* are collectively present in the first complex vowel sound O and the third part is the consonant sound M. The fourth part is the moment of silence that occurs after we have finished chanting *oṁ* and the sound has just left our lips. Each of these audible sounds reflects one of the major cycles or components of the universe, our bodies, the world, and our states of consciousness. And each of these sounds is presided over by one of the principal aspects of the great triumvirate within yogic mythology: Brahmā (Brahma), Viṣṇu (Vishnu), and Śiva (Shiva). Therefore:

Brahmā presides over the A sound.
Viṣṇu presides over the U sound.
Maheśvara (Śiva) presides over the M sound.

Together, these three divine aspects (which are explained in more detail in the Guru Mantra, page 33) represent the cosmic cycle. The last part, silence, represents the complete resolution or transcendence of that cycle, when we've moved beyond it to the state of cosmic oneness or unity.

Oṁ (ॐ) lays its roots in the language of Sanskrit. The sound appears within many traditions, however, both in the East and in the West, through sacred sounds like "shalom" and "amen."[1] It is said that the ancient seers, called *ṛṣi*, sat in elevated states of meditation and heard within their own heart this powerful vibration. Their best estimation of its audible sound was that of *oṁ*. They held that this was the fundamental vibration of the universe. Thousands of years later, scientists have discovered something called "cosmic microwave background radiation" — an all-pervasive vibration that is the earliest remnant of the Big Bang that blankets the entire universe.[2] This seems to confirm the original theories of the *ṛṣi* that vibration is at the source and heart of all things. We see this reflected in many mythologies that describe the world originating with a sound or word. In fact, modern science calls the origination of the universe the *Big Bang*. Once again, sound is at the heart of all things.

Meanwhile, some scientific theories of the universe propose that tiny vibrating strings are the basic building blocks of even the tiniest particles. Whether we look at elemental strings, the strings of a cello, or our heartstrings, all of us are moved in some way by vibration. Vibration is how we measure our brain waves, our heart waves, and our feelings about someone else when we catch their "vibe." While vibrations vary in frequency, if we were to dial them all back into a common resonance, the ancient yogis would say that this basic wave would feel and sound like *oṁ*, or the resonance of the sound within our hearts. When we chant *oṁ* in a large group, the quality of the room will change, as well as the quality of our mind, because *oṁ* has the power to act like a cosmic reset button. It brings out-of-sync vibrations back into sync. It harmonizes the space — in the room, in our heart, and in our mind.

And we like harmony.

Harmony speaks to balance. Balance is what we seek, sometimes at great cost. When our bodies are out of balance, we go to great lengths to restore it — in the case of a fever, for example. When we feel like we're falling, our whole body structure will react to compensate and try to restore balance. Balance can be synonymous with peace and the feeling of being at ease. *Oṁ* does this for us in one easy syllable. Its power is intrinsic, and the word that describes *oṁ* in the Yoga Sutra (1.27) is *praṇava*, meaning "ever new." This indicates the fact that *oṁ*'s power never fades no matter how dispersed our universe and no matter the span of time. This one great syllable carries within it the seeds of all universal potential. While that may sound outlandish, consider the outlandish moment of the Big Bang: everything within our universe was encapsulated in this tiny seed — infinite potential — that then exploded in a cosmic burst, whose residual tone we replicate with this one infinite sound.

2. Guru Mantra

This chant, originally found within the Guru Gītā — a treatise on the importance of the guru — speaks to the essential wisdom every spiritual practitioner must know about the guru.

गुरुर्ब्रह्मा गुरुर्विष्णु
गुरुर्देवो महेश्वरः।
गुरुः साक्षात्परब्रह्मा
तस्मै श्री गुरुवे नमः॥

gurur brahmā gurur viṣṇu
gurur devo maheśvara
guruḥ sākṣāt parambrahmā
tasmai śrī gurave namaḥ

The guru is Brahmā, the guru is Viṣṇu,
The guru is Śiva [Devo Maheśvara].
The guru is nearby and the guru is everywhere.
To the guru, I offer all that I AM.

Advice for Chanting

This is a wonderful mantra for setting the tone of a student's mind-set. It is a great mantra to chant at the beginning of a practice to get into the vibe of learning and be open to new information. As such, this mantra can be used as an invocation for daily practice to keep a "beginner's mind," in practice and beyond, or it can be chanted at the start of a yoga class to encourage students to remain open to all the teachers who are present in their life.

To begin chanting, move through it one line at a time. Say *gurur brahmā gurur viṣṇu,* and move line by line from there. If teaching it to others, use a call-and-response method, going line by line, in order to make the pieces easier to remember and follow along. The last line, *tasmai śrī gurave namaḥ,* can be repeated several times. This brings home the intention of the chant to offer all that we are to the power of the teachers who are present in every form all around us.

The Sacred Relationship to the Guru

This mantra honors the most sacred relationship in yoga, that between the teacher (*guru* in Sanskrit) and the student (*śiṣya*). Indeed, only through the transmission from teacher to student has the Vedic tradition been passed down through the millennia. But more importantly, this relationship contains the power to reveal the most fundamental and basic teaching, which is that we are all connected.

The mantra begins by naming the holy triumvirate of yogic mythology — Brahmā, Viṣṇu, and Śiva — who are the primary teaching forces within our lives. They are the gurus to whom everyone is a student. In the scope of a lifetime, these aspects appear to us in varied forms and lessons. The mantra also indicates that there is something beyond the beyond (*parambrahmā*) — indescribable — to which we are all intimately connected. Though indescribable and beyond our grasp, we can find this force within everything that appears near to us (*sākṣāt*). In this way, the guru appears to us in every form imaginable. Teachings show up within the circumstances of our birth and our parents, which is the realm of Brahmā. They appear in our life through our friends, colleagues, and social duty, in the realm of Viṣṇu. They accompany us through sickness and challenges as we face the end of all things and our own death, or the realm of Śiva. The principle of the guru is always nearby (*sākṣāt*), and it is beyond the expressible forms of the universe (*parambrahmā*).

Some spiritual aspirants find one teacher who leads them down the spiritual path, but all aspirants have a guru present at every moment of their lives, if we have the presence and openness of mind to see it. When someone challenges our moral sensibilities, when our parents invite us over for Thanksgiving dinner, or when our boss withholds a raise we feel we deserve, each of these moments holds an opportunity for us to see one of these guru aspects at work within our lives. We are able to recognize that within every single instant there is a chance to learn and grow.

The spiritual life is lived every moment of every day and arises as a practice in each and every choice we make. It doesn't take yoga pants and mala beads to make someone a spiritual aspirant. It takes the tenacity of spirit and the presence of mind to consistently rise to every occasion and practice one's spiritual calling, which is the unfoldment of the potentiality of one's own soul. Like the knights of the Arthurian grail legends, each of us carves our very own path through the thickets of our internal landscape as we make our way into the deep inner recesses of the heart. There, we discover the treasure of our spiritual path: the guru within, who is the ever-present guide of the heart showing us the way to our own source of freedom. As we walk on this path, moment by moment, choice by choice, we offer all our efforts to this internal and eternal source of wisdom within us. In this way, no matter what stage of life we are in, we are never lost.

A Life Lived in Three Stages

Every single one of us experiences the same three basic stages of life: birth, life, and death. These three stages are certain for every person on the planet, and the triumvirate of Brahmā, Viṣṇu, and Śiva preside over them, respectively. The gurus of birth, life, and death show us the value and lessons within the circle of life.

These three stages are found within every aspect of the universe. The universe itself had a birth, it will sustain itself for a period of time, and then it will die. This great cycle is reflective of all experiences in life — friendships, jobs, homes, families, income. Things begin, they last for a duration no one can predict, and then they end. Sadly, nothing lasts forever. This sentiment can be a blessing (when things are bad) or a curse (when things are good and we hope they'll last). What do we do to exist comfortably within such a tumultuous, inevitable cycle of existence?

We use mythology to give us context and understanding of this inevitable pattern of constant flux. Mythology provides us with a container within which to place the challenging experiences of our lives. Otherwise, we can have difficulty coming to grips with them. The trick is to pay attention to the mythology as it unfolds within us and within the events of our lives. We can use these associations to understand the great wisdom of the time-tested Persian proverb, "And this too shall pass."

Brahmā: The Birth of Our World

Brahmā is the god of creation, and he presides over beginnings and our birth. Funny thing is, we actually have little control over these principles. As babies, our birth is a haphazard experience beyond our control. We come into this life with a prearranged set of parents and circumstances. Interestingly, Brahmā reflects this heir-apparent attitude with his own story. Commonly, it is said that he is self-born within a lotus that sprouts from the belly button of Viṣṇu, and from his four faces Brahmā utters each of the four sounds of *oṁ* (ॐ), which begins the creation of the universe.[3] Another story says that he was born of a great golden cosmic egg that was floating around in the nothingness of numinosity. Again, he is almost self-generated without rhyme or reason. His job is to create the rest of existence, and he begins by creating ten sons from his mind, who help him design and construct the universe. When he feels lonely, he creates his beautiful daughter, the goddess Sarasvatī (Saraswati), by thinking the most pure thoughts possible. Each of his four faces represents the supreme knowledge of the four books of the Veda, and he carries no weapons because, for him, there is nothing to destroy, only unlimited potential to create.

In fact, for us, our birth is a great mystery. We can't remember it personally, except as a story told by others. We are thrust into this life like the mere thought of Brahmā, filled with unlimited potential. As children, all things are possible for us, or so we believe. When asked what we want to be when we grow up, we say doctor, lawyer, astronaut, ballerina, firefighter — anything we want. In our childhood, the world is our oyster. Like Brahmā, we believe we can create whatever our mind conjures.

But then something funny happens. We grow up, and the constraints and confines of society close in around us. We are fettered with the chains of "should" and "should not," and filled with doubt instead of promise. We see that our minds do not make "reality," which in fact makes its own demands upon us.

We may come to feel small, weak, and incapable. Strange how, as we get bigger, the box we live in becomes smaller and smaller.

Harken back to childhood. Remember the dream that kept you awake at night and inspired imaginary play with friends? That dream and that child still lives within and is waiting to be reborn. The dreams of youth are profound, but the problem is that we cannot realize those dreams when we are young. We must reconcile our potential with the constraints of adulthood. We can only follow the path of our unlimited childlike wonder after we have broken out of the chains of immaturity. Given this seemingly unfair setup, it's no wonder that there aren't very many temples of worship specifically for Brahmā in India. He's recognized as an equal ruler in the great triumvirate, and he is often included in common rites, but it is very rare to specifically worship him or seek his guidance. Because, in fact, what can we do to reconcile our birth and beginning except learn to live the experience as a fully conscious adult? And so, we turn to Viṣṇu, the preserving force of life.

Viṣṇu: The Preserving Force of the Universe

Viṣṇu, as the preserving force of the universe, is the energy that maintains every aspect of the duration of our lives. His energy is present in our current relationships, our dynamics at work, and the personal growth we seek through spiritual practice. He is also abundantly present in anything that keeps us moving along. Any time we are in our "status quo," Viṣṇu is there helping us to maintain it. And though he's always present, his job isn't rigorously creative like Brahmā or as creatively destructive as Śiva, and so he is often depicted at rest on his great serpent-couch, Ananta, in the great cosmic ocean of potential. We can imagine this scene: a blissful god lounging in an endless pool on a floaty device with a subtle grin on his face. Though it seems that Viṣṇu is doing little in this idyllic setting, he is hard at work dreaming, and his dreams become our waking reality. When god dreams, anything can happen. And sometimes wild and crazy things stir up the world so much that disaster strikes and we can't quite handle reality on our own.

When this happens, Viṣṇu will incarnate and arrive on earth as a cosmic assistant (called an *avatāra*) ready to lend a helping hand to humanity. Any time the world is suffering from too much strife and sorrow, Viṣṇu will appear in bodily form and assist us back onto the path of dharma, or "duty." Dharma exemplifies the way in which we express ourselves in the world. In a sense, it's our life purpose. Therefore, Viṣṇu represents both the challenges that humans face as adults in the world as well as the source of fortitude and courage to meet those challenges successfully.

In the Puranic tradition of India, Viṣṇu has had at least ten incarnations, including as a fish, a tortoise, a dwarf, and several different men. Probably the most popular of Viṣṇu's *avatāra* is his incarnation as Kṛṣṇa (Krishna), the blue-skinned flute-playing charmer who spends his youth herding cows in the bucolic lands of Vṛndāvana (Vrindavan).

Kṛṣṇa's early life reads like a storybook. In the afternoons, after the cows have come home, he plays his flute in order to round up the cowgirls, with whom he dances into the night. But, like all of us, eventually Kṛṣṇa grows up and gets a real job. Youth makes way for the harsh reality of day-to-day life. His real job finds him driving a chariot into battle with the greatest warrior in the land, known as Arjuna. During his employment, he helps Arjuna overcome his doubt (which becomes the dialogue of the Bhagavad Gītā). Eventually Kṛṣṇa retires to hang out with his one hundred wives (that's hard work!) and best friend, Uddhava.

Even Kṛṣṇa apparently once admitted to his best friend that, in order to be incarnate within a human body, he could only be as much as 15/16 perfect.[4] Without that 1/16 of imperfection, his divine stature would lose hold of its human form. So, from a divine perspective, humanity is almost by definition imperfect. This is our great challenge, and it is also our great gift. Ultimately, meeting this challenge is the source of our own redemption. This happens when we accept our imperfections in order to behold the deeper truth of the greatness of our souls. And, though yogic wisdom tells us that our soul is timeless, as humans we still fear what happens at the end: our death.

Śiva: The God of Death and Dissolution

The third aspect of this life-encompassing mantra is embodied by Śiva, the god of death and dissolution. His realm includes every sort of ending, from relationships and ideas to illness and physical death. Śiva is often vilified for this destructive role within the trinity. His incarnation is often portrayed with matted dreadlocks, scantily clothed, and covered in ash. He makes it his business to meditate like a true mendicant on top of a mountain in the Himalayas in order to realize the nature of reality, which is yoga, or union between the highest self and the numinous. The mythologies describe Śiva as the primordial yogi, at ease with the changeable nature of the universe, as he's the deliverer of its end. That must make change easy for him, as one cannot be attached to something that one knows will inevitably die!

Of course, many people, particularly in the West, are not that comfortable with death. We don't like to see it, and we don't like to think about it. For many, aging itself becomes hard to contemplate, and some people try to avoid the appearance of aging at all costs. Other cultures embrace death and keep it in the forefront of daily life and ritual. For example, in India and in

Bali, extravagant cremation ceremonies can last for days, even months, as people enact rituals that help them to celebrate the life and death of their loved ones.

Known as Maheśvara, the great lord Śiva is often treated like an unwelcome guest. But death is an integral part of life. Further, Śiva presides over the fires of transformation. With utter compassion, Śiva's destruction clears a path for new possibilities and creates the space where anything can arise. Within us, Śiva can help to clear out old paradigms and belief systems to allow what is embedded deeply within our hearts and unconscious to rise to the surface. His energy can move through our life like a forest fire through the brush. Though undeniably destructive, it is also essential for providing the opportunity for new growth.

The Unwelcome Guest

There once lived an old woman who had a dedicated spiritual practice to Lord Śiva. Daily, she would pray to Śiva and make offerings to him on her altar. In the quiet moments she would chant to herself Śiva's favorite song, "*Oṁ namaḥ śivāya*," and always had him at the forefront of her mind. She lived a meager existence and had very little, but she was happy in her simple devotional practices, which kept her busy every day.

One Sunday afternoon, it was time for her to go to the market, and so she gathered her shopping basket and headed off. She always went later in the day because the vendors would price their wares more cheaply and would be more apt to bargain. The woman had very little money and had to be very careful about what she purchased each week, as it would have to last. She made her way through the market, collecting the few items she needed for the week, and as she strolled past the fruit vendor, she spied a perfectly ripe mango set off on the side of the cart. Its ripeness was such that one more day would put it over the edge, but at this very moment, it was at its perfect peak. The vendor saw the old woman eyeing the mango and said, "Is this your favorite fruit?"

"Why, yes, it is, but I so rarely get the chance to have it." The old woman licked her lips after speaking.

The fruit vendor took pity on the old woman and handed her the mango saying, "Here you go, old woman. Please enjoy it. I cannot sell it tomorrow as it will be overripe, and you are the last person here today. Take it as my gift."

The old woman was overjoyed at his kindness and took the mango, carefully placing it in her basket. She walked home smiling to herself at the dessert she would enjoy that evening. Upon returning home, she set out her groceries and prepared a stew that would last her for the week. She added a few spices and some rice to thicken it up. When she was done, she poured a little bowl for herself and ate it, all the while staring at the mango. At the end of her meal, she cut the mango, but at the last minute, decided only to eat half. It was such a rare treat, that she set the second half aside for the next day, so that she could prolong her joy. She said her nightly prayers to Śiva and went to bed.

In the middle of the night, the woman was awoken by a knock at the door. At this time, in this place, rules of hospitality were paramount, so she got out of bed, put on her slippers, and answered the door. A very old, hunchbacked man with a cane stood before her.

"Hello, old woman! I'm sorry to bother you so late, but I have been walking very far and need a place to rest. Could I come in?" The old man shuffled past the woman as she opened the door a little more widely for him to pass. He looked around her tiny cottage and said, "My, my, it smells delicious in here!

What were you cooking? Might I have some? I am so hungry and have traveled for so long." The old woman obliged him and filled a bowl with her stew. She sat across the kitchen table from him and watched him slurp up his soup, while some dribbled into his long, white beard. When he was finished with his first bowl, he asked for another. And then another. After finishing his third bowl of stew — and the entire pot she'd made for the week — he stretched his arms up and surveyed her tiny hut.

"My, what a tidy, quaint place you have here! Oh, goodness, is that a mango I see on your shelf there? It's been so long since I've had one. I sure would love something sweet to follow that delicious meal I've just eaten." The old man patted his belly and smiled at the old woman.

Her heart pitter-pattered in her throat. The mango was her favorite, and she was so looking forward to eating the whole thing. She now regretted not enjoying all of it earlier that evening. As she had these thoughts of lack and selfishness, she caught herself, turned her mind to her beloved Śiva. She quietly said a chant to him and graciously offered the mango to the old man.

He ate it whole in one bite.

The old woman sighed, said another prayer to Śiva in her mind, and smiled at the old man. It was time to go to bed, so she offered him her own meager mattress and found a small spot in a clean, quiet corner for herself. Later, in the middle of the night, the old man startled her by shaking her shoulders saying, "Wake up! Wake up!" She awoke with a start and asked, "What's wrong?"

She looked up at him. Suddenly his features changed and he grew to an enormous stature, throwing off his ragged cloak and revealing his true nature — it was Śiva himself! She recognized him immediately and prostrated before him.

"You bow to no one, old woman. Stand before me and prepare for your journey home." Śiva reached out his pristine hand and lifted her up. She stood with him, hand in hand, and she smiled. He said, "It is because of your consistent devotion and your ability to offer all you have with your whole heart that you are coming with me. Your physical life is over, but your spiritual life is just beginning."

Off they went together, merged as one.

Honoring Śiva Means Letting Go

As Śiva takes the old woman's hand, her lifetime of continuous surrender is what allows her to step into the grace of this deathly

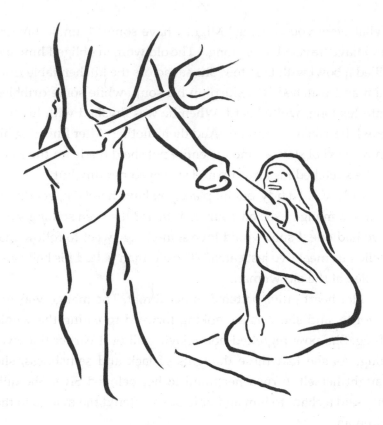

lord. The old woman did not fear death because throughout her life she had consistently shed her expectations and her grip on what life "should be." She let go of little things every day, accepted every "little death," and so when Śiva arrived, she was ready to open herself to him and let go in the ultimate way.

Similarly, honoring Śiva in this mantra is a way of acknowledging this mysterious truth: that when we stop resisting death, and all the inevitable endings we encounter, we step more fully into the timeless flow of life. Death, after all, never truly ends the cycle of life, but is merely the cycle's most transformative moment, for it is the gateway to resurrection. It's like Albert Einstein says: "Energy cannot be created nor destroyed, it can only be changed from one form into another." When we die to our old way of being (whether that includes fear, pride, anger, or resistance), we then shift our energy and open the door for a new way of being (one embodying openness, honesty, integration, and gracefulness). In every mythic story, the hero, like the old woman, must undergo a transformation, which typically involves a death of some kind. In fact, what defines the hero is the willingness to confront fear and doubt and, if necessary, die to overcome the story's challenge. While heroes may have fear, they call forth the courage necessary to overcome it and walk their journey by living from this strength, which resides at the core of their being.

When we live from our own center, even when death touches us, we find courage (literally, the strength of our heart) to face our fear and allow death to bring forth new life. Too many of us ignore death, tragedy, aging, calamity, hard times, and even just the blues, when the secret is acceptance.

The old woman did this in the story. Her entire life was in service of death. She was able to embrace the god of death, Śiva, through her prayers and songs. It allowed her to be at ease with changing circumstances, disappointment, poverty, and personal challenges. It didn't make those challenges go away. It made them *easier to bear*. What if, instead of denying the very real presence of constant change, death, and transformation in our lives, we went forth with courage and used our heart to stay at the calm center of any storm? This is Śiva's gift. This is what he brings to the old woman on the night of her own death: grace through courage.

This release into transformation and the embodiment of acceptance of all the circumstances in our life is also what the last line of this mantra invokes: "To the guru, I offer all that I AM." When we are able to see every moment as an opportunity to be taught and to grow, we give ourselves over to the teacher that is always present all around us.

3. Asato Mā

While the wisdom of the Veda is said to be timeless, its fundamental spiritual ideas have been distilled into shorter bursts of high-powered teachings known as the Upaniṣad. Chock-full of mythological allegories, each of the Upaniṣad illustrates an important tenet of Vedic wisdom. The oldest of these more concise texts is the Bṛhadāraṇyaka Upaniṣad, which gives us an origin tale for the universe that explains how the nothingness became "somethingness" and how our universe further developed into the infinite forms we recognize today. As the universe developed, there also developed the tension between opposites — light and dark, good and evil, knowledge and ignorance. Finding a way to navigate this constant tension is one of the main ways we find solace within our spiritual practice.

The Bṛhadāraṇyaka Upaniṣad probably dates from around 1500 BCE. From it comes this chant:

ॐ असतो मा सद् गमयण
तमसो मा ज्योतिर् गमयण
मृत्योर् मामृतं गमयण

oṁ asato mā sad gamaya
tamaso mā jyotir gamaya
mṛtyor mā amṛtam gamaya

Lead me from untruth to Truth
Lead me from darkness to Light
Lead me from death to Immortality

Advice on Chanting

This mantra makes for a wonderful invocation for practice, or even a silent mantra for meditation. It's a powerful mantra that keeps the aspirant's mind fixed on the issue at hand — moving through the shadows to recognize the light of internal awareness. The beginning of this chant features an *oṁ* that brings to the mantra the initial creative vibration present at the beginning of all things. This relates it back to the source text it derives from, which explains the mythic origins of the universe. In further repetitions of the mantra, the *oṁ* may be skipped in the first line, or it may continue to be chanted. Try moving through the chant one line at a time, and if teaching it to others, use a call-and-response fashion, pausing at the end of each line for respondents to repeat it. Each line contains a pair of opposites — the initial aspect we are moving away from and the complement we are moving toward. The movement between them is expressed by the term *gamaya*. The three lines feature untruth (*asat*) and truth (*sat*), darkness (*tamas*) and light (*jyotir*), and death (*mṛtyor*) and immortality (*amṛtam*). Essentially, for the yoga practitioner, we are always striving toward the light.

Finding Eternity Within Ephemeralness

This invocation from the Bṛhadāraṇyaka Upaniṣad encapsulates a central yogic idea: that there is a source within us that is self-empowered, self-effulgent, and eternal. As humans, we live within the wheel of *saṁsāra*. This is another name for the cycles of life discussed in the Guru Mantra (page 33). As such, each one of us must confront death, ignorance, and error, but we can find our way through this to what is timeless and unchanging. Most importantly, the immortality expressed in this sacred mantra is not the desire for the physical body to live forever. Rather, it's the desire to experience or realize the everlasting source within us — which some call a soul, spirit, *ātman*, or *jīva*.

Further, as the mythic story of this Upaniṣad makes clear, it is mantra and sacred sound that can lead us to this place. Through mantra, and the sacred vibration it harnesses, we can be led home — to our internal, everlasting, self-effulgent essence.

The Cosmic Ocean and the Veil of Manifestation

The universe is sleeping. A cosmic ocean, it lies dormant and quiet. Completely still and absent of light. There is no time or space, just their absence. Lying dormant at the bottom of this ocean of nothingness are millions and billions of tiny seeds, which in and of themselves are also nothing — without time, space, or light. However, within those seeds is *potential*, just as the great banyan tree lies hidden inside its tiny seeds. Those seeds await the proper conditions to sprout. Until then, the seeds remain hidden and quiet. Nothingness ensues.

This yogic origin story — describing a timeless cosmic ocean in which no-thing exists — is equivalent to the scientific origin story of the Big Bang, which proposes that at one point everything in time and space existed as a sort of presingularity…a prepotential state. In Sāṁkhya philosophy,[5] which presents the yogic view, this is known as *puruṣa*, sometimes referred to as consciousness, or unmanifest reality. *Puruṣa* can also be understood as the principle force behind our favorite sound of *oṁ*

— the sound that eventually gives rise to all things, according to Upanishadic and Vedic texts. It's tough to put a finger on the formless, but suffice to say that *puruṣa* is the subtle, underlying source present within all things. It is this potential force that composes this original cosmic soup, without which nothing eventually arises.

Then after a long period — what the tradition refers to as "the night of Brahmā" — creative numinosity begins to stir. Through this indescribable force, the seeds ripen, the atom splits, and suddenly time and space are born. Seeds grow and ripples appear on the surface of the ocean. Waves appear and affect other waves; seeds take root and develop into the fiery element of creation. The power of manifestation, *prāṇaśakti* (*prana shakti*), bursts forth, forming mind, senses, dreams, desires, and eventually the earth or the substance of the universe in all its diversity.

In the story, the manifestations that arise out of the cosmic ocean of *puruṣa* are known as *prakṛti* (*prakriti*), or manifest reality. As *prakṛti* continues to develop and materialize, it becomes denser and denser and further removed — or externalized — from the original source. Eventually, we ourselves become so cloaked in this externalization that we don't recognize the original numinous vibration or *puruṣa* in the things that we see and experience. This cloaking effect (for more on this, see the Gāyatrī Mantra, page 65) is known as *māyā*, or the illusory veil that pulls the world over our eyes so we see and experience only the veil and not the truth that is cloaked behind it.

This is exactly like the concept in the 1999 science fiction film *The Matrix*, in which the hero, Neo, is "unplugged" from the computer simulation that he (and almost everyone else) has mistaken for reality. Through this simulation, humans are kept unconscious of their true plight, as biological energy sources for machines that have taken over the planet. When Neo is first approached within the computer simulation by an awakened man named Morpheus, who is working with others to extract humanity from this dream state, Morpheus must find a way to explain to Neo that what seems to be reality is not actually real. The Matrix, in fact, is a symbolic representation of *māyā*, and the effects of recognizing it as such are the same. Only once we see and understand that everyday reality is *māyā*, an illusion like the computer-simulated Matrix, can we recognize the ultimate truth that lies behind it. In yogic practice, that truth (*sat*) is of our immortality (*amṛtam*). Here is the conversation Morpheus first has with Neo:

> MORPHEUS: The Matrix is everywhere, it is all around us. Even now, in this very room. You can see it when you look out your window, or when you turn on your television. You can feel it when you go to work, or when you go to church, or when you pay your taxes. It is the world that has been pulled over your eyes to blind you from the truth.
>
> NEO: What truth?
>
> MORPHEUS: That you are a slave, Neo. Like everyone else, you were born into bondage, born inside a prison that you cannot smell, taste, or touch. A prison for your mind. Unfortunately, no one can be told what the Matrix is. You have to see it for yourself.

By the film's end, Neo not only realizes that the Matrix is all in his mind, but that his mind is actually more powerful and can control this illusion. This is similar to how we, through yogic practices, eventually are able to see through the veil of *māyā* to recognize the effulgent source (*puruṣa*) at the heart of all things. Once we do, we can control our own reality. We let go of the false understanding that externalized forms are "real" and immutable.

We see past this to the inner reality, which is that timeless, formless, pure consciousness is at the heart of everything.

The Demon War and the Power of Chanting

In the origin story from the Bṛhadāraṇyaka Upaniṣad, the cosmic ocean churns and separates and divides further into the components of the mind, the sensory organs, and eventually the separation of heaven and hell. When this happens, the demons (known as *asura*) and the gods immediately go to war with one another.

And as soon as the demons and gods start fighting, the gods are immediately outdone — there always seem to be more demons than gods! The gods convene to create a plan to defeat the demons through the tremendous power of mantra. Mantra, when chanted correctly, has the power to correct, redirect, and reunify all that is separate. Through its practice, *prakṛti*, or manifest reality, dissolves back into the timeless *puruṣa*. For us, as individuals, this means that mantra has the ability to reunify any feeling of separation we have from our source. This is yoga!

The gods have their answer, their great weapon to defeat the evil demons. And so the mouth, with its grand power of speech, is summoned to chant their chosen words — a chant so powerful and utterly divine that it can harness and channel the power of the universe to overcome evil. But the demons get word of this great plan. They attack the mouth and wound its speech, so that it speaks not just perfect mantra but harmful words as well. The mouth fails, so the gods must find another way.

They enlist the eyes! The beautiful eyes! There is no way for the demons to pierce this beauty, so the gods ask the eyes to chant the sacred mantra. But the demons are clever, and they attack the eyes so that the eyes see not just what is beautiful but what is ugly and fearsome.

So the gods recruit the ears, for perfect ears hear only perfect vibration. The ears chant beautifully until they are pierced by the harsh words of the demons. The ears falter, hearing not only harmonious sound but also cries and screams and terrible untruths. The gods then ask the fingers of touch to learn the chant, for how could touch be spoiled? It is so perfect in its caresses and ability to soothe. But the fingers are pricked and start curling in on themselves, withholding their power and transmitting pain as much as pleasure. The smelling nose is asked to chant, but it is at once overcome with putrefaction and founders.

Well, since the mind thought of this brilliant idea, the gods finally plead with the mind to focus on the perfect chant to help them win this war! The mind focuses intently and is indeed harder for the demons to attack, but once they do, negative thoughts arise and suddenly the mind wonders about its own ability to do this task. Does it even have the skills? Can it do it? Doubt fills the mind, and the mind becomes useless in creating the power needed to overcome the demons.

The gods are heartbroken. They just know that mantra is the only sure way to harness the absolute power of formless, pure consciousness, but how else are they to get to it? All the *indriya*, or organs of action, have failed. But, suddenly, the gods think: "What if it isn't an *indriya* who is chanting? *Indriya* are fallible, as they're made of the divisive nature of *prakṛti*! That's it! We'll enlist the *prāṇa* — the driving force of *puruṣa* — to chant!" And so the gods ask *prāṇa* to chant for them. *Prāṇa* politely and humbly obliges. It begins the chant, not just chanting the mantra, but invoking the very essence of the mantra and driving it forth as the supreme weapon of unification. The demons try and try, but all their attacks are hopeless against the impenetrable, infallible *prāṇa*, whose ultimate connection to the numinous source is indivisible. There is no "other side of the coin" with *prāṇa,* whose nature is unity.

Through *prāṇa*'s embodiment of the mantra, the most powerful weapon — sacred sound — is used to defeat the demons and create peace once again. The gods can rest and finally become what they know themselves to be: perfect, whole, and complete.

The Devil in Disguise

As a mystical practice, yoga allows us to understand the external world on an internal level. In keeping with the hermetic aphorism of Hermes Trismegistus, "as above, so below," the yogi is one who seeks to understand the external world through inquiry into the internal landscape. This means that all life becomes refocused through an internal lens of self-inquiry, where we see that the whole universe is simply a reflection of ourselves. If we understand this myth as a metaphor, then we see that this story of gods and demons is simply an analogy to illustrate our own dualistic tendencies.

As humans we often fall prey to a dualistic concept that makes us feel separate from the source. We allow the tongue to speak harshly, the hands to withhold tender touch, and the mind to rationalize our self-doubt. Yoga, as a mystical practice, involves deep self-inquiry where we travel within to discover where our internal truth, light, and reality reside. The external world shows us our separateness, while the internal world reveals the truth that we are eternally connected to the source of our being.

One of the most powerful methods of focus to help us reveal our internal nature is mantra. As we channel our own energy, or *prāṇa,* into uplifting phrases, then just like the gods, we defeat our inner demons and reveal our own wholeness. Through self-inquiry, we discover the all-connected source within. We stop seeing the external world as "real," and like Neo in *The Matrix*, we discover the ways in which we can reshape and reunderstand ourselves in order to see the world differently. This internal inquiry will reveal the light that is cloaked by self-doubt and self-judgments. People who have discovered this self-effulgence are those who illuminate and inspire others — simply through their presence alone. It is these luminaries who have the capability of transforming the world they live in. And we are all capable of that, for we all come from the same luminescent, vibrational source.

4. Saha Nāvavatu

The relationship between a teacher and student is a major aspect of yoga practice, and within several different Upaniṣad, we find the same mantra, which codifies the ideal nature of this relationship. This version of the chant is found in the Kaṭha, Mandukya, Śvetāśvatara, and Taittirīya Upaniṣad:

स ह नाववतु
स ह नौ भुनक्तु
स ह वीर्यं करवावहै ।
तेजस्वि नावधीतमस्तु
मा विद्विषावहै ॥
ॐ शान्तिः शान्तिः शान्तिः ॥

sa ha nāv avatu
sa ha nau bhunaktu
sa ha vīryaṁ karavāvahai
tejasvi nāv adhītam astu
mā vidviṣāvahai
oṁ śāntiḥ śāntiḥ śāntiḥ

May we both be protected
May we both be nourished by wisdom

May we work together with great energy
May our study be vigorous and effective
May we never experience enmity toward each other
oṁ peace, peace, peace

Advice for Chanting

This mantra is an excellent choice as an invocation for any situation where both a student and teacher are present. The purpose of the mantra is to protect both parties in the relationship and ensure that each is focused on achieving the highest aim within their practice together. The mantra can either be taught by the teacher to the student in a line-by-line, call-and-response fashion, or both teacher and student can chant the mantra together. The end of this mantra includes the simple chant for peace that both teacher and student are encompassing in their work — peace on three levels: personal, mutual, and universal.

The Teacher-Student Relationship

While yoga could be surmised as being all about relationships, it is clear that the most important relationship within yoga is between the teacher and the student. This bond is essential for spiritual growth and has withstood the test of time as the primary mode of dissemination for yogic and Vedic wisdom across five millennia. Only in the past few decades or so has knowledge about yoga become widely available through any resource other than the direct transmission of a teacher or guru. Even so, most modern-day yoga practitioners still get their yoga from teachers. Whether it's the more direct transmission of a one-on-one relationship or the more modern interpretation of a group class setting, we still find most students sitting, listening, and taking in the knowledge of a teacher.

Still, the nature of the relationship is extremely important because it determines the quality of the work and, ultimately, one's success. As this mantra exemplifies, it will ideally be a mutually beneficial relationship. There is no hierarchy or degree of subservience or domination. In fact, this chant is said by both the student and the teacher to clarify their uplifted intentions as they begin working together. In today's world, this timeless mantra is of critical importance.

Teaching in the Good Old Days

The term *upaniṣad* means "to sit near," and the particular grouping of texts that became the Upaniṣad were indeed generally recounted in a story-like fashion, where the student learned directly from a venerable teacher. This was the basic tradition for millennia. Teacher would teach. Student would sit and listen. And through that perfect listening, the wisdom of the teacher would enlighten the student. Literally. This remains a great way to convey teachings, especially in an intimate setting, where the teacher and student can engage in question-and-answer dialogues. This way, the student asks the teacher what they most want to know, and the teacher responds directly and individually.

This is a great system for a few reasons. First, students ask questions only about knowledge they are ready for. This is because, as age-old wisdom tells us, we only ask questions for which we already have the answers. The teacher only reveals what the student suspects already. Second, when a student asks a question, the teacher knows the student is serious about learning. Traditionally, the student must ask three times before the teacher will give the answer. In this way, the teacher can be assured, as Jesus would say, of not throwing pearls to swine (Matthew 7:6).

The practices and the knowledge of yoga were kept pretty

secret for millennia after millennia. There was a good reason for this. It was the care and discernment of the teacher, and their rapport with the student, that helped to direct the teachings in a way that would guide the specific student forward in his or her spiritual endeavors. When teachings are cast in a haphazard, careless way, they may do as much harm as good. Unprepared students may stumble onto teachings that make no sense to them, or worse, are misconstrued. Only a sympathetic, knowledgeable teacher can guide and steer spiritual understanding in a way that is personal, powerful, and appropriate to one's own learning curve.

The Student's Sacrifice

In the Kaṭha Upaniṣad, where we come across this mantra, we also find a classic example of the teacher and student relationship. In the story, a sage performs a particular sacrifice in which he agrees to give away all of his possessions. However, the sage shirks on his promise and only gives away the most spent and aged cows of his herd. The sage's son, Naciketas, is a dedicated student of the holy traditions, and he challenges his father. Naciketas asks him to whom he should be given, since the son is the possession of the father. His dad scoffs and ignores him twice. But, on the third asking, his agitated father finally promises to give young Naciketas to Yāma, the god of death.

Naciketas arrives on death's doorstep and waits for three days. Death is always terribly busy. When Yāma arrives home to find someone waiting for him, which is really never the case, he is surprised and pleased. In his delight, he offers Naciketas three boons — a common tradition among the gods of the yogic pantheon. For his first wish, this bighearted young man asks that Yāma return him safely and alive to his father, and for his father not to be angry with him. His second wish is for the secrets of a fire ceremony that is named for him. Third, and most importantly, Naciketas asks Yāma to reveal to him the secret behind death and the truth of immortality.

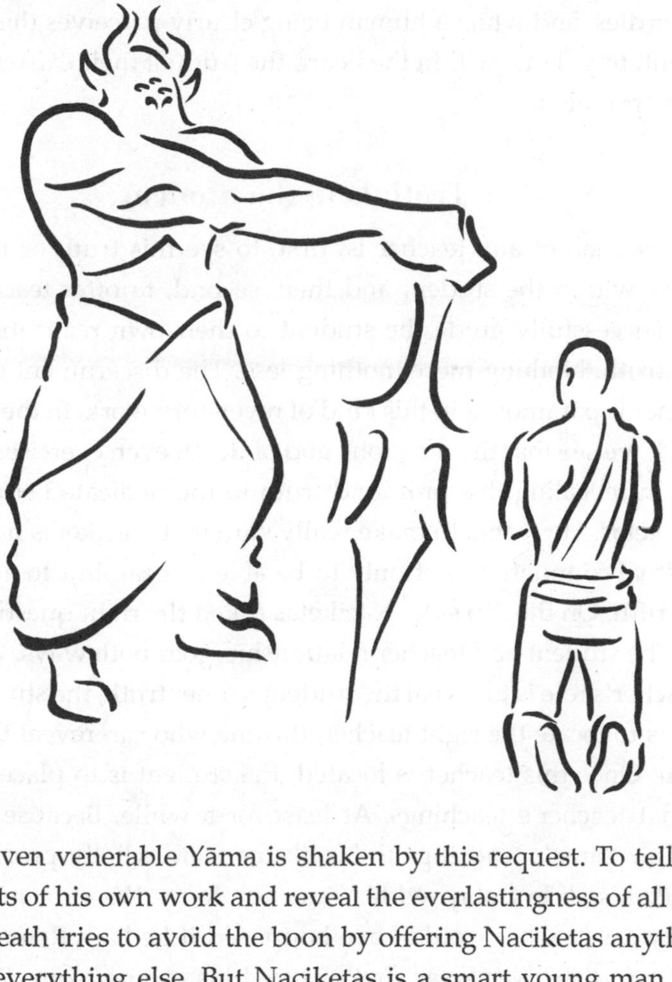

Even venerable Yāma is shaken by this request. To tell the secrets of his own work and reveal the everlastingness of all that is? Death tries to avoid the boon by offering Naciketas anything and everything else. But Naciketas is a smart young man and denies all these offers; he sticks to his guns. He wants the answer to the meaning of life.

Finally, Yāma relents and describes the true nature of the self and its oneness with all things. He reveals that the death of the body is merely an illusion, as the *ātman*, or soul, carries on long after the body is shed. He tells Naciketas that basically his role as Yāma is to reveal the truth of what we truly are: Supreme Source. He informs Naciketas that the soul is never born, and never dies, and when a human being clearly perceives this persistent, tiny flame within the heart, the truth of their existence is verily revealed.

The Truth Is in the Student

The true job of any teacher is, first, to see this truth or numinosity within the student and then, second, to offer teachings that successfully guide the student to their own realization of that truth. Nothing more, nothing less. The discernment of the teacher is paramount in this kind of revelatory work. In the Upaniṣad, we see that the ferocious god of death even exercises caution in revealing this profound truth to the dedicated student, Naciketas. He wants to make really sure that Naciketas has the spiritual foundation, not only to be able to hear, but to absorb the truth. On the flip side, Naciketas asked the right question.

The student and teacher relationship goes both ways. While a teacher's role is to reveal the student's inner truth, the student's role is to locate the right teacher, the one who can reveal this to them. Once this teacher is located, the student is to place faith in that teacher's teachings. At least for a while. Because even though Yāma's teachings to Naciketas were wholly profound, Naciketas didn't stay with Yāma for long. We can surmise pretty easily what would have happened if he had! Remember his first wish? Naciketas first ensured his escape from Yāma's grasp. Without the ability to leave, he'd be lost forever. He never gave his power away to Yāma in their enlightened exchange. He remained the trusting student while hearing Yāma out, and then once the knowledge became his own, Naciketas parted ways with Death, continuing on to lead his own life as a teacher of the truth.

The most important aspect of the precious teacher and student relationship within yoga is summed up by yoga teacher Mark Whitwell,[6] who says, "The guru should be no more than a friend and no less than a friend."

R-E-S-P-E-C-T

The Upanishadic and yogic traditions come from a time and culture that revered the learning relationship. This tradition differs from, and sometimes conflicts with, modern Western society, which places different stresses on the individual to challenge authority and value uniqueness and independence. The clash of this original learning modality with its new setting can result in common problems of imbalances of power. Teachers can find it difficult to establish the right boundaries, so that they can successfully impart wisdom while maintaining the kind of respect necessary to place students on equal footing in the relationship. Meanwhile, students may slip into a kind of subservient reverence for a teacher who seems to have all the answers. As in the above quote, the answer to this struggle lies in the idea that this relationship, while friendly, is not friendship. Friendship is sacred and treasured and exists between two people who can laugh, kid, and challenge each other's ideas. This can be counterproductive in a teacher/student relationship where trust and surrender are key aspects of the student's ability to learn sometimes very challenging, counterintuitive, and difficult teachings. The teacher and student within the context of yoga exists for one purpose: to guide the student home to their highest truth. This setting requires respect between both parties and a certain amount of reverence for the teachings themselves. In our prolific yogic era, we are lucky to have a wide variety of teachers from whom to seek higher wisdom. As students, we have the responsibility to choose our teachers wisely. In both cases, the respect of this relationship will yield great fruit, as it did in the story of Naciketas and Yāma. When Naciketas saw his opportunity to learn, he took it. When Yāma saw his opportunity to teach, he took it. When the teachings had been given and the point driven home, Naciketas made his exit. And this is, perhaps, the most important aspect of the teacher and student relationship.

The teacher's role is to reveal the inner truth of the student's divine self. When that job is done, this relationship must end. This is the final representation of yoga's ultimate goal, which is liberation. It is counterproductive for a student to remain with a teacher beyond the scope of his or her learning. Interestingly, we find a similar concept conveyed by Jesus (in Luke 6:40): "A disciple is not above his teacher, but every disciple who is fully taught will be like his teacher." Once again, internal power is always retained by both parties, as both parties can receive a kind of freedom from this sacred relationship. When the student has received what he or she has come for, then either the student must go willingly or the teacher must set the student free.

Ideally, this occurs when we, as students, learn to stand on our own two spiritual feet. When this happens, we have paid the teacher the greatest honor: we have embodied their lessons and made them our own. The truth lives inside us vibrantly and powerfully in such a way that we come to recognize that the teacher's only work was simply to get us to realize this.

Because, as Yāma told Naciketas, truth resides like a fire, ever-burning, within your own heart. It is ever-present and beyond death. It is who you truly are.

5. Gāyatrī Mantra

The Gāyatrī Mantra is said to be one of the oldest mantras known, and it is thought to be beyond translation. Simply through the repetition of the chant, the deep meaning of the words and vibration eventually resonate throughout the body, effectively changing the consciousness of the chanter. The word *gāyatrī* is a compilation of the roots *ga* (to sing) and *yatri* (protection), and this chant offers protection to our mind as we repeat this sacred series of sounds. This notable chant originates in the Ṛg Veda — the oldest of the four Vedic texts — and is as follows:

ॐ भूर्भुवः स्वः
तत्सवितुर्वरेण्यम्ण
भर्गो देवस्य धीमहि
धियो यो नः प्रचोदयात्भ

oṁ bhūr bhuvaḥ svaḥ
tat savitur vareṇyam
bhargo devasya dhīmahi
dhiyo yo naḥ prachodayāt

Earth, Air, Heavens,
We meditate on Savitṛ, giver of Light,
May he illuminate our Consciousness.

Advice for Chanting

The term *gāyatrī* also defines the specific meter of the chant. Since this mantra is the most famous of that meter, the term has come to refer to this mantra specifically, similar to the way that many of us pair the rhythm of iambic pentameter with the couplets of Shakespeare's *Romeo and Juliet*. The *gāyatrī* meter is traditionally eight syllables per line, but the second line of the chant contains only seven syllables. This indicates that the chanter must offer an extra beat, like a conscious pause, as an act of reverence to the nature of the chant. Typically, this is done in the word *vareṇyam*, by pronouncing it "varen(i)yam." (For help with this meter, listen to the Gāyatrī Mantra audio file at http://alannak.com/musicians-mantras/mantra-library.)

Within the sacred syllables of the Gāyatrī Mantra, we find the sound *dhī* (specifically in the word *dhīmahi*), which is indicative of *buddhi*, or the illuminated consciousness that arises in a state of total awareness. This is the elevated intellect, one that can discern not just between right and wrong, good and bad, but an intelligence that knows there is no right or wrong, good or bad, and that there is only what will lead us toward the light and what will lead us away. The clear power of this illuminated awareness is the ultimate state of consciousness for the yogi — one that will allow swift and consistent progress on the spiritual path.

While this mantra can be chanted anytime, it is perfect set against the backdrop of the rising sun. If your practice has you up that early, try chanting a few rounds of the Gāyatrī Mantra to welcome the sacred light of day.

Savitṛ: The Illuminating Power of Words

This mantra is one of the most notable chants from the Ṛg Veda. Legend says it was written by the great sage Viśvamitra, who began life as a great king and then spent thousands of years in yogic meditation to earn his sage status. At one point, Viśvamitra, who is known both for his extreme anger and his compassion, tried to offer a boon to a student by allowing him to transcend to heaven without leaving his body. Since it was known that those who are ready to enter heaven cannot do so with a physical body (such perfection does not allow one to hold on to human form), he was affronting the laws of nature and the gods. Viśvamitra was disavowed of his sage status, but he earned it back after another several thousand years of intense penance. He is rumored to have penned most of the third *maṇḍala* (section) of the Ṛg Veda, which includes the Gāyatrī Mantra.

This powerful mantra originated in the Vedic tradition of India, in which we find some deities that predate the more modern expression of Hinduism. This includes the primary deity of this chant, Savitṛ. Savitṛ is a solar god who is credited with giving movement to our brightest celestial body. His strength also resides in the great potency of words and utterances. His name is translated as "the magic power of words" by scholar Alain Daniélou,[7] and this reflects the power of sacred sound as the guiding light of creation.

On any given day, before light dawns, everything rests in darkness. And so it goes with us. Before we are moved to brighten the awareness and consciousness of the mind, we are in a state that is known as *avidyā*, or a lack of light. It is the power of the word or speech that calls forth the light from the darkness, just as we find in the mythic cosmology of traditions throughout history and the world. It is the same in the Vedic history, as Savitṛ, the force of the sun, brings the day into being with his magic power of speech. He is said to be one of the primary sons of the great all-mother of the Vedic tradition, Aditi. As a masculine god born from the primordial form (Aditi), Savitṛ helps to negotiate between the realms of humans and nature. And one of the greatest forces of nature, which occurs daily, is the rising and setting of the sun. It is the basis of life on this planet and gives us the construct of time and temperance. The sacred words of the Gāyatrī Mantra are the syllables with which Savitṛ brings this light forward to ignite the life and consciousness of the world.

While the sun has always held a place of significance for human beings, it is also an important symbol. In Eastern traditions, the sun is a metaphor for the light of our own awareness — a measure of our own illuminated consciousness. Without this light, we sit in darkness, *avidyā,* not knowing how to navigate our free movement across the horizon and illuminate the dark reaches of our mind.

Peeling Back the Layers

The source of our illumination, or our internal sun, corresponds to our blissful internal nature, which can be called the *ātman,* or soul, and which is powered by the all-pervading *puruṣa* (for more, see the Asato Mā mantra, page 47). In modern depth-psychological terms, these things correspond generally to the idea of the collective unconscious (*puruṣa*) and the soul or psyche (*ātman*). If we are to mine our darkness to discover the source of our internal light, then we need to work through the layers that are covering over this self-effulgent source. According to the yogic tradition, our body contains more layers than just skin, muscles, and bones. Ultimately, there are five layers, and they can express either the density and heaviness or the lightness and clarity that we embody.

These five layers (or sheaths, *kośa*) are grouped into three "bodies": the causal body, the subtle body, and the gross body. The causal body is made up of the blissful sheath — the *ānandamaya kośa.* The subtle body is composed of the intellectual sheath, the mental sheath, and the physiological sheath — the *vijñānamaya kośa, manomaya kośa,* and *prāṇamaya kośa,* respectively. The gross body or the food body is the *annamaya kośa.* The three bodies reflect the three layers of the world: heavens (causal), air (subtle), and earth (gross). Each person possesses these three bodies, and therefore reflects the external world on an internal level. This understanding is what's referred to in the mystical reading of the Gāyatrī Mantra, which opens by naming "Earth, Air, Heavens."

The earth, air, and heavens are within us, and so is the giver of light. Nestled in the layers of the body and the effulgent self, we have a perfect mystical reflection of the chant, along with the prayer to illuminate the *buddhi* consciousness of perfect discernment (known as *viveka*) that will allow us to lean toward the light as we progress on our spiritual journey.

These sheaths or layers of the body are each made of *māyā,* or the manifest reality that allows us to operate in the world. Like a lampshade over a bulb, they cover over the innermost, luminous self, or *ātman,* which is transcendent of *māyā.* As each layer sheaths the one underneath it, the light of the self becomes dimmer and dimmer until it can no longer be seen by us or anyone around us, and we are cloaked in our own darkness. Through yogic practices, particularly sacred mantra, these layers can be made more transparent, so that our inner light can shine outward like the sun upon the earth. We've seen people who radiate in this way. These are the folks who light up any room they walk into. Their smiles give warmth and brightness, and we feel a little more radiant just by being in their presence. These are the people who are unafraid to let their own light shine.

At our core sits the self, the *ātman*, or the most primal connection to the all-pervading numinous source. It is encapsulated within the first layer, the "blissful layer" or *ānandamaya kośa*. This layer is "blissful" because it is snuggly wrapped around the most connected part of us, the part that knows ourself to be an integrated piece of a much bigger whole. The *ānandamaya kośa* is called the "causal body" because its proximity to the self is what helps to make manifest the rest of our being: when our decisions, choices, and actions are fueled by our soul, then we fully manifest our blissful self in the world. However, this delightful interaction between manifest/unmanifest can be stifled if we are disconnected from the numinous, or if the outer layers are too cluttered and dense to allow this spontaneous, self-directed mode to be put into action. It's like the sun rising on an extraordinarily cloudy day, so that despite its movement across the sky, it can't really be seen.

Wrapped around the *ānandamaya kośa* is the *vijñānamaya kośa*, or intellectual layer. This is the layer that is our personal manifestation of *buddhi* consciousness. As the *prakṛti* (manifest reality) arises from the *puruṣa* (unmanifest reality), the next thing to be manifested is the *buddhi* consciousness. If we think of Buddha as one who has fully expressed *buddhi* consciousness, then we have a model for how this works. An illuminated intellect uses its powers of rationality to discern what will lead us toward the light and what will lead us away. It is important to note that what leads each of us toward the light can differ. There is no one way to walk the spiritual path; there is only the one way that is right for each person. It is our *buddhi* consciousness that guides us precisely and gives clarity to the multitude of decisions we have to make as we march on. If our intellect is dense and dark, then we get bogged down by the monotony of making decisions based on external influences and circumstances, rather than allowing ourselves to make those decisions based on our own internal nature and bliss. The greatest obstacle to the clarity of this layer is boredom, or apathy, as it stifles this enlightened intellectual process.

Next up, we have the *manomaya kośa*, or layer of the mind. This isn't the intellectual mind, but rather the emotional mind — the one that gets caught up in preferences and likes and dislikes and is hell-bent on staying in the comfort zone. Which, incidentally, is a zone that gets smaller and smaller the more attached we are to it. Eventually, we are only comfortable at a specific temperature, with a specific meal, in a specific location, with a specific person. How much suffering we feel when those conditions are not met! Imagine softening these attachments so that no matter what the meal, temperature, or person, we are comfortable and confident in our situation. This layer contains the *ahaṁkāra*, or ego, and is fed by the five senses. It asserts I-ness every chance it gets, making sure that the most important consideration is given to our own desires and attachments. This is sometimes in our best interest. Each of us is a unique and special snowflake that has an idiosyncratic way of interacting with the world — and the world is made better through this color and variety. It is when we become overly attached to our own way of doing things that challenges arise and selfishness sets in. The greatest obstacle to the clarity of this layer is selfishness, but it can be offset by engaging in selfless actions, connecting with others, and interacting with our spirit. For example, dedicating our time to walking shelter dogs and chanting to the different aspects of divinity are two ways of getting us out of our own heads, out of our small comfort zones, and creating more transparency in the *manomaya kośa*.

The next layer operating dynamically within us is the *prāṇamaya kośa* or physiological layer. We could think of this as the moving parts inside our body: the blood, lymph, and nervous systems, our breath and endocrine systems, all interact to comprise this layer. In yogic terminology, this layer is fed and moved by *prāṇa,* the life force that vivifies us and moves through various energetic channels (for more on this, see the Vande Gurūṇām mantra, page 77). The more fluid and malleable we can make our body, the less stuck this *prāṇa* (and indeed, the other bodily systems) will become. Fluid motion is key in this layer, as stagnation leads to injury, illness, or chronic pain. This layer is addressed through energetic practices and most specifically (in yoga) through *āsana* practice, breath work or *prāṇāyāma,* and chanting. All three of these yogic practices are designed to correct and align the energetic pathways so that *prāṇa* can move freely through us. Chanting works subtly but powerfully, and *āsana* makes us work physically to access *prāṇa*'s subtle movement. Because *prāṇāyāma* works directly with the *prāṇa,* it acts like a key in a lock for unleashing energetic clarity.

These three layers — *vijñānamaya, manomaya,* and *prāṇamaya* — make up the subtle body, which is "subtle" because its effects can be felt and experienced but are difficult to translate or quantify. Often, our thoughts, interests, and energetic wellness are a subjective experience that we can't convey to others. We may be able to feel the expressions of these layers, but these personal experiences are hard to physically measure with modern-day instruments. We can measure brain waves, for example, but those waves cannot be read as cogent thoughts. We can measure levels of hormones and chemicals in the body, which may indicate certain types of emotional reactions, but this doesn't reveal the complexity of emotion and thought that triggered them. There are things in our lives that are beyond measure but lived daily. We can agree, objectively, that everyone experiences them, but it is only the subjective experience that allows us to comprehend, explore, and understand the workings of our own bodily structure to attain a sense of inner harmony.

Finally, the last layer is the *annamaya kośa*, or the food body. We've all heard the term "you are what you eat," and that reflects exactly the principle of this layer. The type of food we put into our mouth literally becomes our body. On a simplified level, the heavier and denser the food, the heavier and denser this layer will be. The lighter and more clean the food, the more transparent the *annamaya kośa* will be. This layer is our physical body — the dense "unflowing" parts like the skin, muscles, and bones — and it is our vehicle for this spiritual process. Like changing a car's oil every three thousand miles and making sure we never run out of gas, the way we eat has a big effect on how our bodies carry us along. There is no singular prescription for how to eat for enlightenment, but our body is a vibrant feedback mechanism. When we pay attention to it, it gives us important clues as to the kind of fuel it prefers and runs on best. As we clean up our diet and eat according to our body's needs, we'll find that the physical lightness translates into an ease of being in our body and a confidence that we can feel comfortable with.

Chanting Through the Layers

As our spiritual practice develops, we engage all these layers on a regular basis. *Āsana* helps to create lightness in the physical body and correct imbalances of the physiological body. Meditation can inspire the intellect and engage the mind. *Prāṇāyāma* keeps the mind busy and regulates the movement of *prāṇa*. Every yoga practice plays its part in creating transparency in these layers so the innermost self, or *ātman*, can shine forth brightly. Interestingly, the one practice that has a direct and profound effect on all the layers is the practice of chanting mantra. It is as Sufi mystic Vilayat Inayat Khan says, "In the mantram practices one actually kneads elaborate bundles of nerve fibers that are the plexi or ganglia...are subjected to a consistent hammering....There is a kind of seizure of the flesh by the vibrations of sound."[8]

First of all, mantra is a physical experience (*annamaya kośa*) that recruits the body into feeling the sensations of sound and vibration. We open our mouths to sing, we sit and sway to the beat, we clap our hands, we engage our ears in listening, and we close our eyes to tune in to our internal world. Physiologically (*prāṇamaya kośa*), our breathing is regulated by the singing of the chant, and if we're in a room with other chanters at a kirtan, then our heartbeats fall into sync and match the rhythm of the drums. The chant helps to regulate the flow of *prāṇa* within our body so it can be channeled for the spiritual ascendance of *kuṇḍalinī* — which is explained further in the Vande Gurūṇām mantra (page 77). Our mind (*manomaya kośa*) is focused on something greater than ourselves. When we chant, we're not thinking about our problems, our discomfort, our bad decisions or negative habits. We've stepped outside the confines of a restrictive comfort zone and opened the narrow box we sometimes find ourselves in. Our intellect (*vijñānamaya kośa*) is engaged by the singular focus of the chant, whose aim is to lead us toward the light. Finally, our blissful layer (*ānandamaya kośa*) is most connected to its source as we let the vibration of the numinous reverberate throughout our entire body.

Chanting works like magic.

It illuminates every part of us. It engages all five layers of our three bodies to create transparency so the light of the self can shine brightly through us. As each of these layers becomes more transparent, we're able to harness our internal light and become sources of illumination for those around us. As we do, we bring to life, internally, the meaning and nature of the Gāyatrī Mantra. We let the sun shine through the three abodes of the manifest reality and use the words of the chant like magic prayers to give rise to an illuminated consciousness.

6. Vande Gurūṇām

AṢṬĀṄGA OPENING MANTRA

Yogic wisdom describes an energetic body within all of us that responds very specifically to mantra. (For a description, see the Gāyatrī Mantra, page 65.) Through the wise use of vibration and the application of *nāda* yoga, or sacred sound, we can align ourselves internally and externally to fall into sync with our yogic pursuit: creating the right condition for our inherent state of yoga to arise naturally. The way in which this state arises, metaphorically, within the yogi's body is harkened to in the first part of this composite chant, which traditionally begins the Aṣṭāṅga Vinyāsa (Ashtanga Vinyasa) style of yoga practice. This style was originally taught by Krishnamacharya to Shri K. Pattabhi Jois and was later popularized by Jois's teachings.

This chant is composed of two parts. The first is a verse that comes from the beginning of an eighth-century text called the Yoga Taravāli, which was written by Ādi Śaṅkara, a well-practiced yogi and sage (though his actual dates are in dispute). The second part is a traditional invocation that comes before the chanting of the Yoga Sūtra — probably the most popular and important yogic text — to invoke its legendary author, Patañjali.

वन्दे गुरूणां चरणारविन्दे ।
संदर्शित स्वात्म सुखावबोधे ।
निःश्रेयसे जाङ्गलिकायमाने ।
संसार हालाहा मोशान्त्यै ॥

vande gurūṇām caraṇāravinde
saṁdarśita svātma sukhāvabodhe
niḥśreyase jāṅgalikāyamāne
saṁsāra hālāhala mohaśāntyai

I bow to the lotus feet of the guru
Who awakens the happiness of one's own Self
Just as the snake charmer who removes poison
Reveals the truth behind the illusions that bind us

अबहू पुरुषाकारं
शङ्क चक्रासि धारिणम् ।
सहस्र शिरसं श्वेतम्
प्रणमामि पतञ्जलिम् ॥

abahu puruṣākāraṁ
śaṅka cakrāsi dhāriṇam
sahasra śirasaṁ śvetam
praṇamāmi patañjalim

To he who has realized the Self
And who holds a sword, conch, and discus,
Who is white-headed and crowned with the thousand-
petaled lotus,

To Patañjali, incarnation of the great serpent, I offer all my prayers.

Advice for Chanting

These two mantras are most often now chanted together at the beginning of an Aṣṭāṅga-style yoga class, but they are from two different sources, and they could be chanted separately to invoke different intentions. The first part of the chant from the Yoga Taravāli very clearly focuses the practitioner on the energetic goal of yoga, to awaken *kuṇḍalinī* in order to hear and feel the internal vibration, the *nāda*. If the aim of your practice is to create energetic awareness or sift through any physical or energetic "darkness," then the first part of the chant can be used to focus the mind in that way.

The second part of the chant gives thanks to Patañjali for codifying the wisdom of yoga in the Yoga Sūtra and honors Patañjali in his legendary form, a snake-man. It is an invocation that is traditionally said before embarking upon study of the Yoga Sūtra — a wise idea for anyone serious about the mystical path of yoga. Depending on the aim of your particular practice, feel free to use each stanza on its own. For example, if you have decided to take up a study of the Yoga Sūtra, or are reading a translation of this popular text, try beginning your study by saying the second portion of this chant. It is also appropriate to move through this rather long chant line by line on your own or in a call-and-response fashion.

Kuṇḍalinī: Awakening the Serpent Within

In a story that relates to this chant's first section and its author, Ādi Śaṅkara is said to have once gotten into a debate with a fellow sage and bested him with his knowledge. The fellow sage's wife didn't like seeing her husband defeated, so she challenged Ādi Śaṅkara to a debate on the intimacies of marriage, knowing Ādi Śaṅkara was a practicing celibate priest. However, because of his yogic prowess, Śaṅkara had earned some *siddhi*, or yogic powers, that allowed him to enter the body of a dead king in order to understand how the king...ahem...pleased two wives. Armed with this knowledge, Śaṅkara went back to the wife and bested her in their debate as well.

Ādi Śaṅkara achieved *mahāyogi* (great yogi) status, and the Yoga Taravāli text that he penned reveals important wisdom on the yogic aims, including stages of enlightenment as well as the importance of focusing on internal sound, *nāda*, as a key in the pursuit of the realization of yoga. In order to unlock the cryptic meaning behind the chant's first part, we must understand the metaphorical workings of the subtle anatomy of the body — including *kuṇḍalinī*, the snake who is awakened through the directed force of *prāṇa* — and how sound and vibration play a vital role in the cultivation of an elevated consciousness. Ultimately, this chant is about awakening the potential energy that lives at the base of our spine and that causes us to experience a state of self-realization.

To start, the "snake charmer" in the translated chant is a reference to the guru, or teacher. Sometimes the Sanskrit is translated as "jungle physician." The implication is that this kind of guru is a badass who can remove the poison from even the worst of bites. A snake charmer can draw a sleeping snake out of its hiding place and keep it focused on the sound of his flute. Symbolically, the yogi is aiming to do the same thing with the sleeping serpent inside of him- or herself.

This snake arises out of our energetic body, which was discovered by the *ṛṣi* of long ago in their deep states of meditation (for details, see the Gāyatrī Mantra, page 65). What they learned then was that energy moves within us in specific channels, and when that energy is moved in certain ways through spiritual practice, then it changes our state of consciousness. This realization has parallels in other traditions, including Chinese medicine, Sufism, Native American traditions, and others. In the yogic tradition, energy is referred to as *prāṇa*, which moves throughout the body in channels or rivers, known as *nāḍī*. There are rumored to be 72,000 energetic channels in the body (per the Haṭha Yoga Pradīpikā), but for this discussion we can focus on three main channels: the *iḍā*, the *piṅgalā*, and the *suṣumnā*. The *iḍā nāḍī* begins at the base of the spine on the left side and spirals up the body to terminate at the left nostril. The *piṅgalā nāḍī* begins at the base of the spine on the right side and spirals up the body to terminate at the right nostril. The *suṣumnā nāḍī* begins at the base of the spine and goes up through the center of the body and terminates at the crown of the head. Where these three channels cross, we find a *cakra* (chakra), or an energetic hot spot (these are also the locations of major nerve plexi in the body).

When we do our spiritual practice, we are aligning our energy and allowing knotted or blocked channels (*nāḍī*) to clear up so that our *prāṇa* can move easily throughout our body. Eventually, through diligent practice, our energetic channels become well balanced, and at that time our *prāṇa* begins to move up the *suṣumnā nāḍī*, which can be translated as "ray of light." Symbolically, the *iḍā nāḍī* on the left side corresponds with lunar or feminine energy and involution, while the *piṅgalā nāḍī* on the right side corresponds with solar or masculine energy and revolution. When these oppositional energies are balanced, we are said to be in the process of *haṭha* yoga — which translates directly as the union of sun (*ha*) and moon (*ṭha*). The central channel, *suṣumnā nāḍī*, represents a state of perfect balance between pairs of opposites and a state of evolution.

When we're ready to evolve, it's time to feed the beast.

There's a hungry snake, named *kuṇḍalinī*, who lies dormant and quiet at the base of *suṣumnā nāḍī* until we get the fire of our spiritual practice going and initiate the process of spiritual evolution. *Kuṇḍalinī* is not just a pretty name; it translates as "coil" and represents our own consciousness. Understood to be the feminine principle of śakti (shakti), she is coiled three and a half times at the base of *suṣumnā nāḍī* like a stopper on a tub, not letting anything through until something releases the blockage. Only spiritual intensity can do that. Note that this is not the same as spiritual overkill. We don't awaken *kuṇḍalinī* by practicing forcefully to the exclusion of everything else. The awakening of *kuṇḍalinī* is a mark of the balance of all dualities: inner and outer, left and right, sun and moon, playtime and practice. When *kuṇḍalinī* senses that our spiritual life's direction is heading toward the evolution of our inner and outer lives, then she begins to rise up the central channel, going through the levels of consciousness present at each of the seven chakras.[9] As we evolve we don't "get over" problems or conditions, as if they were suddenly passé, but rather we gain an elevated or evolved perspective on problems as both integral and integrated parts of our life.

This is the way of the jungle physician — or the snake charmer. Take your pick. We essentially become the snake charmer cum physician as we rid ourselves of the poison of delusion. We are sick with ignorance (*avidyā*), and as we remove this poison through practice, we gain the clarity of spiritual awareness and allow *kuṇḍalinī* consciousness to rise. The snake is charmed into ascending up the ladder of consciousness. We then feel an energetic shift as we move about our day. We receive more internal clues about how to make decisions about what best serves our highest good. Because our energy is focused on spiritual evolution, we see clearly what uplifts us and allows for an elevated state of mind. This is the mark of having the poison removed. This is the gift of the guru that is asked for in the last line of the chant, who "reveals the truth behind the illusions that bind us."

Through this teaching of the removal of ignorance, the ascension of consciousness, and the arousing of the subtle energetic body, we can become "joyfully awakened" (*sukhāvabodhe*). In this process, we become our own snake charmers and realize the importance of the quiet hiss of the internal sound that is the *nāda*, the driving force behind spiritual practice and the awakening of spiritual consciousness.

Patañjali: The Great Serpent

The second part of the chant is an invocation that honors Patañjali, regarded as a half-snake, half-man incarnation of the great serpent Ananta, who sits with Viṣṇu as he dreams the world (see the Guru Mantra, page 33). Not much is known about who the real Patañjali may actually have been. Whether he was only one person or is a conflation of multiple people, he is said to have compiled the Yoga Sūtra sometime around 200 CE. The Yoga Sūtra is a summary text that in less than two hundred verses contains the entire body of yogic wisdom packed into short, terse, memorable phrases that are like skeleton keys for a deeper understanding of yoga. The Yoga Sūtra is the most popular resource for yogic wisdom, and many teachers (in both the East and the West) have sought its breadth of compacted knowledge for pearls on the spiritual path.

In the translation of this mantra, Patañjali is described holding three highly symbolic items: a sword, a conch, and a discus. The discus is a gift from Viṣṇu, and it is called the *cakra*, which internally represents our energetic centers, or chakras,

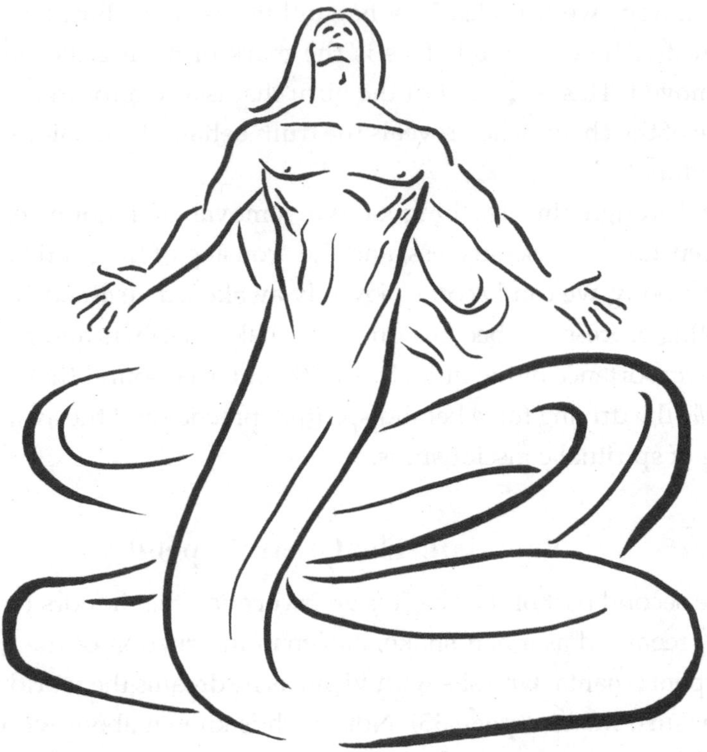

but mythologically, it is a weapon that can cut through anything — particularly ignorance of the true self. The conch contains the power of the all-pervading sound of *oṁ*, which is the fundamental vibration of the numinous source. The sword he holds represents discrimination (*viveka*) — the ability to tell what will lead toward the light and what will lead away. Like Sir Lancelot crossing the harrowing sword bridge to reach Guinevere in the tale of "The Knight of the Cart" in Arthurian legends,[10] the sword is a sharp edge that painstakingly delineates what will serve us and what won't…and what won't gets cut away.

The top of Patañjali's head is said to be both white (or pure) and crowned with a thousand-petaled lotus (*sahasra* in the transliteration). This is also the name and description of the crown *cakra* (chakra) and the symbolic indicator of one whose *kuṇḍalinī* has awakened and ascended all seven levels to exist at the highest level of consciousness. Symbolized in world mythology as the halo, the *sahasra* is a crown of light that signifies one has taken on the spiritual and inner work necessary to shine brightly from the inside out. It seems Patañjali is quite the snake charmer and jungle physician himself!

He was, so much so that through his own yogic perfection he was able to craft and compile the Yoga Sūtra in order to help many students achieve the same kind of spiritual mastery. Within the text of the Yoga Sūtra, Patañjali weaves the entire fabric of yoga together with short threads, or *sūtra,* that shed light on our path so that we may illuminate ourselves. Each aphorism is a gem that demystifies one aspect of yoga. Each gem of a *sūtra* reflects in such a way that, at first, the gem's shininess may be difficult to catch. But with consistent studies, we will eventually come to see the way that these gems shine within ourselves. After all, the jungle physician isn't out there coming to rescue us from the poisons of the world. Rather, he has left clues for us to clear away the poison and become our own snake charmer and jungle physician. Patañjali left us these gems to show us that the power of yoga is within, and so that we can discover own illuminated consciousness and reveal our own halo-crowned nature.

7. Lokāḥ Samastāḥ

AṢṬĀṄGA CLOSING MANTRA

If any mantra were to embody the spirit of the yogi, it would be the closing chant of the Aṣṭāṅga Vinyāsa (Ashtanga Vinyasa) yoga practice (the system of yoga *āsana* popularized by Shri K. Pattabhi Jois), in particular, the last line: *lokāḥ samastāḥ sukhino bhavantu* ("May all the world be equally happy").

Though this chant is rumored to have originated in the Veda, its exact placement within the text is unknown. It is clearly an important mantra, though. It appears in several other circumstances to impart blessings, including at the end of an abridged version of a text known as the Sundara Kandam, which is a story devoted exclusively to the monkey god, Hanuman.

स्वस्ति प्रजाभ्यः परिपाल यन्तम्
न्यायेन मार्गेण महीं महीशाः ।
गो ब्रामणेभ्यः शुभमस्तु नित्यं
लोकाः समस्ताः सुखिनो भवन्तु ॥

svasti prajābhyaḥ paripāla yantam
nyāyena mārgeṇa mahīṁ mahīśāḥ
go brāmaṇebhyaḥ śubham astu nityaṁ
lokāḥ samastāḥ sukhino bhavantu

May everyone on earth know happiness and well-being.
May the protectors of the earth do so with justice and virtue.
May never-ending joy bless those who understand the true nature of the world.
May all the world be equally happy.

Advice for Chanting

At the end of an Aṣṭāṅga Vinyāsa yoga class, you are likely to hear this chant. Sometimes the teacher will chant it on his or her own in order to bless the students, and sometimes the students will chant along with the teacher. It is appropriate to use this chant in any circumstance to impart good will and blessings. Try learning this chant line by line, or teach this chant in a call-and-response fashion to students. Interestingly, the last line of this chant has become something of an anthem for the yoga community, and it is not at all uncommon for only the last line of this mantra to be used as a chant or kind of prayer on its own.

Basically, the last line of this mantra wishes for equality and happiness for everyone everywhere, without any kind of theology or hidden agenda involved, which makes it a wonderful, universal expression of beneficence. This shorter chant is sometimes given a more flowery translation, but the simplicity of the call of these four words really need no dressing up to impart their eloquent message:

lokāḥ: location (everywhere)
samastāḥ: sameness or equality
sukhino: sweetness or happiness
bhavantu: unto all

Hanuman and Humility

With this chant, we wish for everyone to enjoy the same happiness and equality, without any further qualifications or demarcations. It's a universal mantra that asks us to disregard any judgments of others related to their social status, ethnicity, nationality, religion, or spiritual practice. Everyone is born with a right to happiness and equality, and essentially it's up to us to do our part to make that happen...particularly when we see disequilibrium or oppression taking place.

While this chant is rumored to have originated in the Veda, it is also found as a closing prayer in a shortened version of the Sundara Kandam, which is the fifth book of the Rāmāyana devoted exclusively to the monkey god, Hanuman. Because Hanuman embodies a heroic openheartedness and works tirelessly throughout the tale to uplift others, he is a fantastic representation of the essence of this chant. It's no wonder that the chant is used at the end of a text dedicated to the monkey deity who had a hand in restoring peace to the world! Hanuman is the best friend of King Rāma and serves him faithfully throughout the adventures of the Rāmāyana (for more, see the Śrī Rām Jai Rām mantra, page 133). Hanuman's youth, however, was fraught with challenges and ill judgment. Some may have even called Hanuman a bully! Hard to imagine when we hear of the heralded monkey god as the one who leapt across an ocean to save his best friend's girl.[11] But even the best of monkeys have to learn how to be humble somehow.

In one version of the tale of Hanuman's younger years, his demigod status earned him more trouble than it did praise. He was born without fear, and this caused a terrible lack of judgment and pompousness. While playing in the woods, he would chase after deer and pull them by their tails. He would smash trees and pull them up by their roots. In the hermitages of the *ṛṣi*, he would steal their meditation cushions and jump through the trees with them, and he would pull on their beards as they sat blissfully in concentration. His poor behavior was mostly overlooked because the *ṛṣi* knew that Hanuman was an incarnation of Śiva, and that his purpose in this lifetime would be to serve King Rāma and help restore prosperity, happiness, and justice to the land. But this incorrigible boy was just too much to bear.

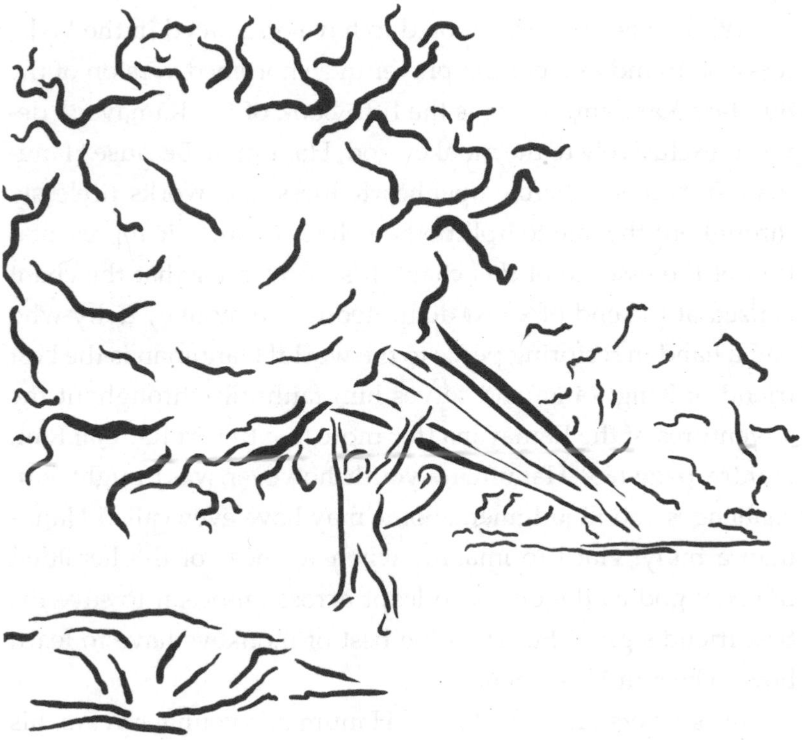

One day, Hanuman's mother went to the *ṛṣi* in the hopes of enrolling him in their school so he could be well educated. They shared with her his unkind actions, and she was shocked. After some discussion, they decided upon a plan. They would make Hanuman forget his powers. If he couldn't remember his demigod status, his pompousness would subside, and in its place, humility would arise. Humility is the number one quality of a yogi, the sages knew. And, with this quality, Hanuman would be able to complete his academic studies and eventually become one of the most eloquent, intelligent monkeys around. Not to mention, his ability to serve Rāma would be heightened, as humility is what allows for service to others and attention to their needs. Later, it is only when Hanuman is reminded of his greatness, during adventures with his best friend, Rāma, that he remembers what great treasure lies inside of him.

The Practice of Cultivating Compassion

This mantra asks for blessings, protection, and happiness for all, but those things don't necessarily appear just because we ask for them. We must cultivate compassion within ourselves in order to be the kind of person who actually *brings* those things to the world around us. This task is made easier through the priceless quality of humility. Interestingly, both the words *humble* and *human* have the same etymological root in Latin: *humus*, which means "close to the earth." As a monkey, Hanuman was by nature a forest creature. But as an incarnation of Śiva, and one whose father is the wind god Vayu, Hanuman sometimes felt he was above others. He forgot his earthly roots and connections, causing him to disrupt the lives of others in a harmful way. Forgetting his demigod status brought him back down to earth, and his story is one of notable compassion and kindness toward those he loved most.

But did he really forget his divinity?

In an interesting twist, it was the forgetting of his godlike status that allowed him to embody his true inner nature. By the end of the tale, Hanuman has become undoubtedly the favorite of the people. They know his big heart is filled with nothing but love and a deep connection to his beloved friend Rāma. It is this connection that inspires Hanuman to move mountains, raise the (nearly) dead, and build a bridge that spans an ocean. Hanuman isn't showing off. His actions embody his devotion and love for his best friend. This complete faith in the contents of his heart (in Sanskrit called *śraddhā*) becomes his most godlike quality. But to manifest this divine quality, he had to forget he was god.

This is different from destroying the god within. This is also different from negating any notion of god. Rather, this story asks us to consider what consumes the majority of our energy. To what do we devote ourselves? Do we spend most of our energy in prayer, devoted to a notion of divinity? Do we spend most of our energy gossiping on social media? Do we spend most of our energy frustrated with how our life has turned out? Whatever we pour our energy into — be it anger, the Internet, or divinity by any of its many names — these form the altars to which we bow.

If, like Hanuman before the *ṛṣi* made him forget his divine status, the only god we pray to is our own ego, then we suffer from hubris — the state of inflation that, in Greek mythology, led to punishment by the Olympian gods. Psychologically, hubris will always lead to a smack down of some kind. Whether externally or internally, the tower we've built to prop up our ego will come tumbling down sooner or later.

Then we'll be back on the ground, right back where we came from. When we maintain a close connection to the earth, to humility, to our humanness, we remain connected and compassionate toward others. Connection and compassion are essential qualities for leading a well-balanced and well-adjusted human life. When we chant, these qualities are also what give power to the mantra: *lokāḥ samastāḥ sukhino bhavantu*. The mantra comes true because we're invested in making it true — we recognize that it's up to us to treat everyone as an equal, as just as deserving of happiness as we are.

Hanuman's lesson is a good template for our own life. His forgetfulness is not a curse but a remedy for the ills of disconnection. We are all divine by birth, but like Hanuman, we often become disconnected with our highest self. For us, the remedy becomes forgetting about our ego and choosing humility in order to cultivate connection to our fellow earth dwellers. No matter what god we prostrate to — even if it's one of a different name, or of no name at all, whatever we deify within our life becomes magnified. Like Hanuman, it is through our acts of love that we reflect the godlike face of compassion and humility. So build your altars wisely and pray to the things that will bring peace, happiness, and equality for all.

8. Oṁ Namo Bhagavate Vasudevāya

Children have a lot to teach us. From the value of play and imagination, to the focus they can cultivate when they find something that matters to them, to the love that seems to ooze from their pores from dawn to dusk, children are a vibrant source of spiritual teachings. One child in particular within yogic mythology holds special status, as does the mantra he uses to cultivate the highest spiritual wisdom. He is Dhruva, and his story is found in both the Bhagavata Purāṇa (the text on the mythology of Kṛṣṇa) and the Viṣṇu Purāṇa (the text on the mythology of Viṣṇu). His mantra is simple, and it focuses on finding the greatest love imaginable, the love that we all seek, which is located within our heart. Through this mantra's repetition, Dhruva earned a place among the stars.

ॐ नमो भगवते वसुदेवाय ॥

oṁ namo bhagavate vasudevāya

I sing the praises of the name of God, the son of Vasudeva!

Advice for Chanting

As in Dhruva's story below, this mantra is perfect to repeat many times as often as you feel inspired. Because it is short, this mantra lends itself well to chanting in a kirtan-type fashion, but it can also be chanted silently as part of a focused meditation practice.

Dhruva: Praising the Proper King

In the mantra, Dhruva praises the "son of Vasudeva." This is a reference to Kṛṣṇa, who is an incarnation of Viṣṇu. For Dhruva, and for us, this is the only chant we need to ascend to the heavens.

As the mythic story goes, King Uttānapāda had two wives. His first wife, Sunīti, had a son named Dhruva who was not favored by the king. As it turned out, however, his second wife, Queen Suruci, who was a beautiful but jealous woman, wanted her son, Uttama, on the throne. So Suruci manipulated her husband into overlooking Dhruva and even denying him any affection. But five-year-old boys are very persistent, and so little Dhruva one day ran to his father and leapt up onto his lap, pushing his brother, Uttama, out of the way. While sitting on his lap, Dhruva smiled up at King Uttānapāda, who did not even look at him or hold him. Queen Suruci saw Dhruva upon Uttānapāda's lap and sneered at him.

"What do you think you're doing, you rotten little child? Do you think you'll ever be loved by your father? No! Your worst deed was to be born of your mother, and because of that, you will never sit on the throne. The best you could ever hope for is to win the favor of the godly father, Viṣṇu. But good luck with that, because even people who try for many lifetimes can't win Viṣṇu's supreme love." With that, Suruci scooped Dhruva up and threw him out of the palace.

He and his mother were sent packing, and on the road, as Dhruva was crying, he recounted the awful tale to his mom.

Sunīti, a good-hearted but meek woman, listened to her distraught son. When he was finished, he asked her, "Mama, is it true? Will no father love me? Not Uttānapāda? Not Viṣṇu?"

His mother felt helpless to do anything about Uttānapāda, so she thought for a moment and replied, "Well, I've heard that Viṣṇu is actually very loving and may hear your prayers if you promise to say them every night." Thinking she was instilling a good habit and sense of faith in her boy, she was glad at her response, though she had no idea how seriously he would take her suggestion. The next morning, little five-year-old Dhruva, whose name translates as "willpower," had all his things packed in a knapsack and informed his mother that he would be leaving.

"Where do you think you're going, young man?" his mother asked, with her hands on her hips.

"I'm heading into the forest to pay penance to Viṣṇu. If I can't have the love of my father here on earth, then I want to get the love of the father in heaven. If I can't ever be king of this world, I want to become king of all the worlds!" He walked away from his mother, who was too stunned to stop him. She did follow him far enough to see that he'd found a spot in the forest right in the center of the seven holiest meditating *ṛṣi*, so she knew at least he'd be safe and protected.

With that, Dhruva got down to business. Serious business.

He sat in his perfect *āsana*, or seat, on the ground, day and night. Not stopping for rest or food, Dhruva performed incredible austerities and intense concentration, until he was noticed by the great sage and celestial minstrel, Nārada. Nārada came to him and asked him why in the world a boy so young would be doing such intense yoga.

"Because I want to be king of all the worlds and earn the love of the heavenly father, Viṣṇu," Dhruva astutely replied.

Nārada was pretty impressed. He'd seen some ascetics in his day, but never one so young. He decided to throw the kid a bone.

"Look, little man. You really want to get into Viṣṇu's good graces? Then say his name. There isn't any sound in the world that anyone likes more than the sound of their own name. Here, I'll teach you the best chant ever for that: *oṁ namo bhagavate vasudevāya*. Say that three times a day — morning, noon, and night — and you'll for sure come to know Viṣṇu's love, and that it springs from the center of your own heart."

Dhruva was psyched. He started chanting and meditating on the mantra. Along with sacred offerings and rituals, his days were spent consumed with the divine chant and his attention to the love of Viṣṇu. He became so preoccupied with his yoga practice that one day, while standing on one leg, deep in meditation, one hemisphere of the earth sank under his big toe. That, coupled with the fact that his ridiculously still breathing began to choke the earth and heavens, made some of the gods start to panic. They weren't sure what to do with the little boy, so they thought they could trick him.

Indra, the so-called manager of the heavens, came to him disguised as Dhruva's mother, Sunīti, and begged him to come home to her, to stop all this nonsense yoga practice and go back to being a kid again. He wasn't fooled by this, nor was he moved by the plea. The gods sent the demons to attack Dhruva, but his hard work had earned him cosmic protection from his attackers, and he stood fast. Finally, the gods went to plead with Viṣṇu himself.

Indra said, "Lord Viṣṇu, look, this kid is doing this crazy penance in your name, and we all think you should go stop him. He's disturbing the balance of the worlds!"

Viṣṇu was intrigued and decided to check on the spiritual

progress of the young boy himself. He went to the forest, stood before Dhruva, and called his name, but the boy did not move. He was so lost in contemplation that he kept his eyes closed in order to hold the inner vision of Viṣṇu within his heart. Finally, Viṣṇu decided he would trick him, and so he removed the vision from the young boy's mind. Dumbfounded, the boy opened his eyes to see reflected before him the same image he saw within.

Dhruva immediately dropped to the ground in prostration. His heart nearly burst out of his chest with his love for Viṣṇu. Viṣṇu returned the favor.

"Young man, never in all the ages of the world have I seen such intense devotion, and certainly never in one so young! You have earned whatever it is your little heart desires."

Dhruva was so overcome by his emotions and delight that he was unable to eloquently say any words. Viṣṇu placed his conch shell (the symbol of *oṁ*) next to Dhruva's cheek, immediately imparting to him the power of speech. With this, Dhruva immediately began to say the most eloquent praises of Viṣṇu the world had ever heard. When he was finished, he finally asked for what he wanted, which was to be the king of the world.

"Certainly, you will be!" said Viṣṇu. "And, not only will you become king of this world, but when you are finished with that post, I shall appoint you as the king of all the worlds. You will become the polestar around which all the heavens turn. In this way, you will look over the three worlds: earth, space, and heavens. And all the worlds will look up to you for guidance of the body and spirit."

With this pronouncement, Dhruva finally returned home. As he left the presence of Viṣṇu, he was struck with doubt over his request. He thought to himself, "How stupid was I? I could have asked Viṣṇu for anything, and I chose to ask for material glory and prosperity in the form of a kingship? How bothered was I by my stepmother's words that I still wanted my worldly achievements after all this penance? This is so ridiculous. I should have just asked for liberation from this life, so that I could ascend to the heavenly abode immediately."

Nārada sensed his disturbance and came to the aid and support of his young friend. While walking beside him, he said, "Look, little man, don't be so hard on yourself. You are so young, and yet you have achieved in only months what it takes most people lifetimes to achieve! But the fact is, you haven't even lived a lifetime yet. Go. Enjoy this one. And enjoy it with your elevated consciousness knowing all the while that it is fleeting and so very precious."

Dhruva liked this advice and resolved to make it a good life and to be the most enlightened king he could be. He no longer worried about seeking approval from his earthly father because he knew that he had found the greatest love that there is in the universe — the love that resides inside the heart. He knew that no matter where he went, how old he got, or how his life would play out, that if he ever needed love, he had only to look within his own heart.

Finding True North

Dhruva's story landed him among the stars, and indeed, the polestar became his heavenly abode, just as Viṣṇu promised. The seven sages that accompanied him in the forest during his meditations became the constellation that we know of as the Pleiades — which, in the Vedic tradition, is known as the Saptarishi or "seven sages." They, and the whole rest of the sky, turn around him. His intense focus on the source of Viṣṇu's love within his own heart became the fixed point around which his life turned, and so it is Dhruva that is the fixed point around which we turn.

His story and spirit are a great symbol for us to follow because we are all looking for guidance.

In some form or another, we are looking for a fixed compass that will always point to true north. Like the polestar around which all the heavens turn, our own guidepost is the fixed point within our heart that is the center of our own being. Sages and saints have come to know this through the practices of mysticism, and for some of us, it takes a very long time to understand that the refuge we seek is within. What if, just what if, it wasn't actually that hard?

What if instead of trying to earn some type of spiritual merit, we were content with the spirit we were equipped with? This is the difference between the path of effort and the path of grace. One includes attachments. The other does not. Letting go of our attachments is not always easy. But there's one approach that may make the task a little easier. We can become like a child. Children are notoriously carefree. They focus on play. They satisfy their basic needs quickly and then move on to their creative urges. They're proud to show off their work and excited to get their hands dirty. They look upon the world with new eyes because they're seeing it for the first time. They are largely unfettered by the kinds of responsibility and attachments that bog adults down in the daily habits and doldrums of so-called life.

Spiritual leaders like the Buddha and Jesus consistently recommend releasing earthly attachments in order to attain spiritual truth. For example, in the Book of Matthew (19:24), Jesus says, "It is easier for a camel to pass through the eye of a needle than for a rich man to enter the kingdom of god." Jesus also recommends adopting the innocence of childhood, for, "unless you become like children, you can't enter the kingdom of God" (Matthew 18:3).

That doesn't mean we must abandon our lives and meditate nonstop in the forest like Dhruva. Rather, we can take the story's lesson to heart and remember to regard our life with childlike wonder. To appreciate and savor it because it is wonderful. All the parts of it. The bumps and the bruises are like badges of honor. The twists and the turns are nimbly navigated by the young at heart. The challenges become like a game to play and win. We may take the game seriously, but it is fleeting.

Though we have responsibilities, we need not take all of those responsibilities out of context and make them the fulcrum around which our life turns. Dhruva was serious about his spiritual practice, and it is probably because he was unfettered by the trappings of adulthood that he was able to commit to the practices of a sage. When, in the end, he realized the spirit of the life-giving force within his heart, he came to realize that the heaven he sought was not just among the stars. It was also right here on earth. Because the road to heaven must be heaven. Otherwise, you're on the wrong road.

9. Oṁ Tryambakaṁ

The liberation mantra known as Oṁ Tryambakaṁ, or the Mṛtyuṁjaya Mantra, comes to us from a tantric text known as the Mahānirvāṇa Tantra. It is traditionally chanted in order to overcome any kind of ailment or restriction — which pretty much makes it appropriate for nearly any situation! Ultimately, the kind of ailment we're looking to overcome is the sickness of *avidyā,* or the ignorance of ourselves as anything other than purely divine and self-effulgent. The kind of restriction we're looking to overcome is the bondage and drama of our life, and that liberation is called *mokṣa*.

ॐ त्र्यम्भकं यजामहे
सुगन्धिं पुष्टि वर्धनम् ।
उर्वारुकवि बन्धनं
मृत्योमुक्षिय मामृतं ॥

oṁ tryambakaṁ yajāmahe
sugandhiṁ puṣṭi vardhanam
urvārukam iva bandhanaṁ
mṛtyor mukṣiya mā amṛtat

> We bow to the three-eyed one, who is fragrant and supremely nourishing and represents the supreme Light of inner wisdom. May we be released from all bondage and suffering just as the stalk gently releases the cucumber. May our minds be overtaken by this supreme Light, which is the immortal nectar of Śiva.

Advice for Chanting

This mantra is heralded for its healing properties — whether you want to heal an illness of the body or the mind. It is also a great mantra to use when something has ended, whether it be a relationship or the life of someone close to you. This mantra expresses a desire for freedom or release from something that needs to be shed, so it can also be used as a "birthday" mantra to celebrate the release of the old year and the hope for something new and fresh in the next.

In all the mantras in this book, the translation of Sanskrit words into English is rarely directly one-to-one. However, translations of this mantra take more grammatical liberties than usual, otherwise it would be unintelligible. For this reason, I haven't tried to match the line breaks in the original Sanskrit. When learning this mantra, going line by line will help make the memorization of the whole stanza easier, and it can be taught to others in a call-and-response fashion. Eventually, chanting the whole mantra and repeating it will help focus the mind on the freedom it seeks.

Candra: Healing the Lunacy of Love

The Oṁ Tryambakaṁ mantra gives praise to Śiva as the three-eyed one, meaning, one who has the ability to see beyond any false illusions. It talks about *puṣṭi,* or a sense of fullness that appears to be almost self-evident, or self-nourished — as when a cucumber becomes so nourished by its parent stalk that it falls from it. This refers to the release from any kind of bondage or ailment, but in particular it is the release to immortality, which is a state of *mokṣa*, or enlightenment.

Until we get to that point, there are many little ailments and restrictions that this mantra can be helpful in overcoming. It is designed to restore health, to elevate our awareness to our center of higher consciousness at our third eye, and to provide protection from any negativity. It was originally given as a healing mantra for the moon, Candra (Chandra), so that he would be protected by the powerful god Śiva.

As Candra, the moon is imagined as a powerful force who presides over the mind and emotions. He is a grand figure whose chariot is drawn by ten white horses nightly across the sky. But the moon is a changeable force whose heart is a fickle lover. Once, while churning the ocean of milk in an attempt to make an elixir of immortality, Candra nearly blinded the gods who created him, so he was immediately banished to the outer atmospheres. From his far-off residence, he became known for his ability to provide romantic lighting and for the gift of divine nectar, which often appears in the form of morning dew.

In one story, because of his nightly parade, Candra is noticed by the great king Dakṣa, who offers his lovely daughters, known as the Nakṣatra, as wives for Candra. There are twenty-seven young ladies in this group, and Dakṣa requests that Candra love them all equally. Candra promises Dakṣa that they'll all have an equal place in his heart, and so the Nakṣatra sisters follow Candra into the night sky. Each one of the lovely ladies takes up her post as a bright star along the ecliptic plane through which the moon traverses on his nightly journey in the heavens.

There is one gorgeous star, however, that the illustrious

charmer Candra cannot seem to stay away from. She's a little bit brighter than most of the others in the sky, and she blushes every time she sees the moon. The beautiful Rohiṇī (which in Western cultures is the star Aldeberan) captures Candra's heart, and he spends most of his nights with her, dancing in the sky. Her sisters become quite jealous of this preferential treatment; they are left to their own devices with no additional illumination in the darkness. Their loneliness turns to rage, and they go to their father, King Dakṣa, to complain. Well, what father can resist the pleas of twenty-six lovely daughters? He hears them all out and then calls a meeting with Candra. Candra arrives at Dakṣa's doorstep full of luster, beaming with love. He smiles proudly and extends his hand to Dakṣa in greeting. But instead of a warm welcome, Dakṣa curses Candra, fating him to whither away. Candra is immediately struck and begins to lose his shine. Little by little, every day, Candra's brightness fades as he wanes into the darkness. Before his light goes out completely, he seeks help from his friend Śiva. If anyone can help him in this time of crisis, it's the mighty lord Śiva, who is the remover of calamities, the restorer of fullness, and the liberator from death.

Knowing the drama that is occurring between her father and Candra, Dakṣa's youngest daughter, Sati, also comes to Candra's aid. She has long been a fierce admirer of Śiva, and Sati teaches Candra a special mantra — the Oṁ Tryambakaṁ mantra — in honor of Śiva that will allow Candra to prove that he is worthy of the great Śiva's assistance. Through reciting this sacred prayer, Candra wins Śiva's favor, and Śiva offers Candra refuge high up in his hair, where Candra can drink the *amṛtam*, or nectar of immortality, any time Candra's form wanes too much. This special drink restores Candra slowly to his fullness over a period of time.

With lessons learned and refuge given, Candra is returned

to his post in the sky, where he traverses across the ecliptic spending each night among one of the shining Nakṣatra, not favoring one more than the others. The curse still stands, however, and he still must garner help from Śiva as he goes through his monthly cycle of waxing and waning. Today, we can see the close relationship between Candra and Śiva, this great bearer of nourishment and healing, any time we look at an image of Śiva and see the moon residing in Śiva's great dreadlocked tresses.

Reflections of the Mind

Humans have long had a grand love affair with the moon. We chart our lives around it. In many cases, it has an actual pull on our life and body cycles. The moon has been associated with "lunacy" or craziness, and it is thought that the full and new moons possess particular holds on our psyche. Metaphorically, the moon is associated with the mind, which is changeable and only reflective of the light of the sun, unable to produce its own illumination. We can think of our phases of life in terms of the moon's phases, beginning with our birth at the new moon, and the first quarter being the dawn of adolescence, the full moon being the turning point of adulthood, and the last quarter being the shift as we prepare for death.[12] These lunar cycles and rites of passage reflect both an inner and outer story. It is a power that has a great hold over every one of our lives.

In Sanskrit, the term for this kind of hold is *graha*. It literally means "to grip." As we see with the story of Candra, even he is fazed by the grasp of his own pull. His emotions and mind draw him to one bright star at the slight of the others. His story involves a sublimation of power to the mighty Śiva as he realizes he needs support on his journey. And, finally, he is restored to fullness, only to begin the cycle again. This is quite reflective of the phases of our mind, and it's the reason why this particular mantra is so very helpful for overcoming the powerful fluctuations of the mind.

No matter how focused we may be on our spiritual practice, our thoughts and attention are still swayed. Though we may think we are on our way to enlightenment, we've still got to do the laundry. Our life goes on, and often we get pulled, just like the gripping tide, into the drama and story of our so-called reality. We fall in and out of love, we fall in and out of trouble, and we fall in and out of health. We rise up like the ocean when things are going smoothly, and we crash like breaking waves on a rock when things fall apart. No matter who we are, or where we are, or in what time we are living, our lives are reflective of the moon's lunatic state and the changeable nature of its reflective light.

What if we had a remedy to change all that? What if we had a tool for understanding and unlocking this grip — to become free of it? For now, we work with this mantra. We can repeat it and embody its underlying message to overcome smaller ailments and restrictions. It can be like a medicine for us when we have a different kind of headache, the kind where our thoughts are running wild and heading into that downward spiral we have all experienced. As the mantra works its way deeper into our system, and we systematically root out some of these layers of bondage — to our career, our relationships, our ailments, our human condition, and our negative self-images — we see things differently. We basically shift the lens through which we look at the world, which makes the world appear completely different to us.

And a miracle is simply a shift in perception.

The miracle that occurs when we step out from this occlusion is that we see that we are not reflective beings, as the moon is, but that we are the self-effulgent ones. Joseph Campbell, in his comparisons of life to the phases of the moon, talks about a critical shift that can occur only at the point of fullness. During the stage of the full moon — which, astrologically speaking, is the point at which the full moon and the self-luminous sun are found at exactly opposite but equivalent positions in the sky — the full moon and the sun appear to be equal in size and luminosity to each other. They are each a shining reflection of the other. Metaphorically, this is a stage of fullness where we feel so nourished by our internal resources that we understand ourselves to be the only answer to our problems.

When we are ready to take responsibility for our lives, our condition, and our awareness — when we become unafraid to say "yes!" to life and face it head on — then we are no longer pulled or gripped by the moon. We then make the leap from the reflective condition of the moon to the self-effulgent, fully aware condition of the sun, which represents full conscious awareness, or the state of *mokṣa*, or liberation.

As the mantra says, we become free of all calamities and bondage. We know ourselves as Śiva, in this regard. We are the ones who can offer nourishment and light to those around us. We hold the moon in our hair, just above us, and we are rarely touched or swayed by drama and emotion. They are still a part of our lives — we walk around with them and hang out with them daily — but the forever-light of the sun resides in our heart. We become free.

10. The Three Mahāvakyas

In virtually all of Vedic wisdom, the ultimate goal is to realize the source of one's internal nature. While this is said in slightly different ways, it's like looking at variations of species of butterfly — all of which fly on beautiful wings, though the colors may express themselves differently. The yogic philosophical and mythological model is one of an internalized, mysticized nature, where the focus is turned within to find the source of our being, no matter what name we give to it. In fact, a popular phrase, and one of the most notable lines of the Ṛg Veda, is *ekaṁ sad vipro bahudhā vadanti*, or "The Truth is one, though the sages call it by many names."

In the millennia-old Vedic texts, the idea of the internal source of truth — a notion that encompasses the numinous source — is encapsulated in three distinct sayings. The first, *tat tvam asi*, is found originally within the Sama Veda and is repeated in the Chāndogya Upaniṣad. The second, *aham brahmāsmi*, comes originally from the Yajur Veda and is also found in the Bṛhadāraṇyaka Upaniṣad. The third, *so'ham*, is found originally in the Īśa Upaniṣad. As with a clever teacher, Vedic texts drive the same point home by repeating it over and over again.

तत्त्वमसि ।
tat tvam asi
Thou art That

अहम्ब्रह्मास्मि ।
aham brahmāsmi
I am Brahman

सोऽहम् ।
so'ham
I am It

Advice for Chanting

Each of these three "great sayings," or *mahāvakyas*, are special in that they are said to be the simplest version of the truth, which is that we are essentially the numinous source of our being. As such, they can be said as quick reminders when we are in a moment of doubt or forgetfulness, or they can be used as part of a larger, more focused meditation or chanting practice.

The third mantra, *so'ham*, is a contraction of the phrase *śiva aham*. The Sanskrit *aham* means "I am," and *śiva*, in this case, represents our highest self (see the Oṁ Namaḥ Śivāya mantra, page 181). Known as the *ajapa* mantra, or silent mantra, this mantra is built into our inhalation and exhalation. If we listen closely, we can hear the quiet hiss of the "sssooooo" on the inhale and the "hhhhaaaammmm" on the exhale, particularly if we amplify the breath through *ujjāyī* breathing by slightly constricting the back of our throat, almost as if we are imitating Darth Vader as we breathe. This constant internal *so'ham* is like a reminder to the mind to remain attached to the still point of consciousness, which directs us to the source of our being.

The Unpronounceable Sound Within

The most important point of the teachings rooted in the Vedic tradition is that the essential source, the unexplainable mystery, lies within. Like a great drop from the mighty ocean, each of us has inside an element of the numinous. Though the Vedic tradition cloaks the numinous with many different multifaceted deities, all these images are simply masks of god, so to speak. The all-pervasive source described within the Vedic tradition is unknowable, unnamable, and undilutable — no tongue has ever soiled it and no words can ever describe it. As soon as we try to put thought forms around it, it is suddenly lost, like trying to look directly at a bright star in the night sky. One must look slightly away in order for the eye to catch the brightness of its light, which was sent to us long ago. So really, we are only seeing evidence of that star's existence, just as we find evidence of the existence of the numinous through its many different aspects.

Rather than getting wrapped up in the various terms for "god," which reflect our cultural and individual perspectives, with the help of these *mahāvakya* chants we can focus on the essence of what the many varied terms for god point to, which is beyond thought, precedes words, and is found within. These *mahāvakya* of the Vedic tradition suggest that everything we need to know is inside, rather than outside us in the form of an expert or a canon filled with rules and regulations. In the Bṛhadāraṇyaka Upaniṣad, the phrase *aham brahmāsmi* is used to explain this concept further as the "great unborn that dwells within the lotus of the heart."[13] This particular *mahāvakya* encourages us to let go of all outer trappings, to shed the fetters of all that is not the source of inner truth, in a method of spiritual negation (illustrated by the famous phrase *neti-neti*, "not this, not this"). When we're thus stripped down, rather than seeking outward for the source of our own being, we focus inward to find the source of empowerment. This notion of the self-as-source is embodied in clear and concise ways with all three *mahāvakya* mantras.

Each of these mantras can be used to still the mind, which is said to be like a cobra being charmed by the snake charmer. Normally, the cobra is a dangerous animal, driven only by primal instincts, just as the mind (particularly the ego) is also driven by primal instincts and will do anything to preserve itself. The ego can be tamed through the one-pointed focus of the mind, which helps to keep the wild, errant thoughts at bay. As the cobra focuses on the sound of the snake charmer's flute, the ego is captivated by the sound of the breath (as with the *so'ham* mantra). This is a primary entry point into the sacred practice of *nāda* yoga, which leads one to the source of the sacred sound that is said to flow from the heart.

Through focusing the breath, the mind will come to know the power of the highest truth, which resides in the heart. Long have spiritual traditions pointed to the heart as the internal location of the source of being. And while we might concede that every atom within our body is alive with the life-giving source (and that every atom everywhere is alive with it, too), many of us experience the measure of our highest, most connected experiences from the heart. Not only is this a lived experience for many of us, this is also reflected in the wisdom of the Veda and other various yogic scriptures that tell us that the all-pervasive sound of *oṁ* (ॐ), the *nāda*, lies inside the abode of our heart.

Thou Art That

The chant *tat tvam asi* comes from the Chāndogya Upaniṣad, which is one of the oldest principle Upaniṣad. It primarily deals with the realization of the self and the fact that the source lies within the heart of all things. One of the first lines of this

Upaniṣad tells us that, "*oṁ* is the Self of all."[14] We are once again pointed to the nature of the source as all-pervading vibration. In the eloquent words of Joachim-Ernst Berendt, from his book *The World Is Sound: Nada Brahma*:

> The world is sound. Not: the world is vibration. Of course, one could say that as well — it is true, and everybody says so. But it isn't precise enough. From the standpoint of physics, there are billions of different possible vibrations. But the cosmos — the universe — chooses from these billions of possibilities with overwhelming preference for those few thousand vibrations that make harmonic sense.[15]

If ever we were to wonder "What is the nature of the all-pervading source?," we have the answer from a multitude of mythologies that the most consistent quality of the numinous is sound. No wonder mantra works so well to connect us with that! Sacred sound can give us direct access to the source, and the Chāndogya Upaniṣad confirms this for us in a later line by saying, "Side by side, those who know the self and those who know it not do the same thing; but it is not the same: the act done with knowledge, with inner awareness and faith, grows in power. That, in a word, tells the significance of *oṁ* (ॐ), the indivisible."[16] What is it to know the highest self? The wisdom of the Chāndogya Upaniṣad tells us through a tale of a father and son that to know the self, to feel the vibration of the numinous as it exists within us and around us, is to know that we are that: *tat tvam asi*.

Śvetaketu's Great Lesson

As the story goes, Śvetaketu was Uddālaka's son, and when he came of age, his father told him that it was time to study with a venerated teacher because the spiritual life is important to explore. Śvetaketu went off to study with a teacher for twelve long years. During this time he learned the wisdom of the Veda, and he became very pleased with his intellectual knowledge of the spirit. But it is not enough to know about the spirit. One must come to know the spirit for oneself, as one's self.

When Śvetaketu arrived home to his father, his father asked what he'd learned. Śvetaketu began to wax poetic about the wisdom of the sages and recite perfectly memorized lines from the Veda. His father shook his head and asked, "Did they not teach you the most basic of all the teachings? Did you not come to know the truth about the great spiritual wisdom? Though you are prideful of your knowledge, did you not ask your teacher about what will allow you to listen for that which cannot be heard?" Uddālaka then began to explain in simple terms the prevalence of the numinous within. He explained that it is like playing with a lump of clay, and so coming to know all things that are made from clay. Or it is like a bird on a tether that eventually settles on a branch, as the ego eventually settles into the highest self. Or it is like salt, that when placed in a bowl of water, cannot then be removed, but pervades and changes the water because of its dispersed presence. At the end of every metaphor, Uddālaka tells Śvetaketu, "Thou art that," *tat tvam asi*.

In the translation by Eknath Easwaran, we find a gem from this part of the Chāndogya Upaniṣad:

> In the beginning was only Being, One without a second. Out of this was brought forth the cosmos and entered into everything in it. There is nothing that does not come from it. Of everything, it is the inmost Self. It is the truth; it is the Self supreme. *tat tvam asi*.[17]

That's pretty much it. 'Nuff said. What we seek is within.

11. Oṁ Pūrṇam Adaḥ

This revered chant is the opening invocation to the Īśa Upaniṣad, which often stands at the beginning of a collection of principle Upaniṣad. The number of Upaniṣad varies according to whom you ask, but generally, it is agreed upon that there are 108 Upaniṣad, of which 18 are the principle Upaniṣad, and Īśa leads the way for the rest of them. With only eighteen verses, this short Upaniṣad conveys an essential element of condensed Vedic wisdom, and the opening invocation is an even more refined, clear version of the ideas contained therein. In fact, Gandhi said, "If all the Upanishads and all other scriptures happened all of a sudden to be reduced to ashes, and if only the first verse in the Īśa Upaniṣad were left…[the Vedic tradition] would live forever."[18]

ॐ पूर्णमदः पूर्णम दिम्
पूर्णात्पूर्णमुदच्यते ।
पूर्णस्य पूर्णमादाय
पूर्णमेवावशिष्यते ॥

oṁ pūrṇam adaḥ pūrṇam idam
pūrṇāt pūrṇam udacyate
pūrṇasya pūrṇam ādāya
pūrṇam evāvaśiṣyate

That is completely whole. This is completely whole.
From the completely whole, the whole arises.
Even when the whole is negated,
what remains is still the completely whole.

Advice for Chanting

This chant revolves around the concept of the word *pūrṇam*. While this word is often translated as "whole," as we'll see below, there are multiple ways to consider this translation and its meaning for us as practitioners. Because of its multiple meanings, this chant has many purposes within our practice. It is, as always, appropriate to chant this line by line or to use it as a mantra for silent meditation. The popularity of this chant has even caused it to be used by some modern-day kirtan practitioners as a call-and-response chant, once again enforcing the idea that there are few rules and many exceptions within this ecstatic tradition.

Pūrṇa: Everything and Nothing

The musician and performer Dave Stringer has pointed out that if this chant were an equation, this is what it would look like:

$0 + 0 = 0$

And

$0 - 0 = 0$

The word we find repeated in this mantra is *pūrṇa*, which is translated as full, whole, or complete. But, in the fullness, we become empty. We become absent of any ideology, desire, or suffering. In our completeness, we know ourselves to be missing nothing, and so we are no-thing, devoid of this or that, up or down, right or wrong. *Pūrṇa* is an idea that encompasses everything and nothing, fullness and emptiness, because these are actually parallel concepts. Zero is both the absence of everything and the presence of infinite potential. Its rounded shape conveys a circular idea of completeness with no end and no beginning. No matter whether we add, subtract, multiply, or divide it, it is always equivalent to itself. This is a beautiful concept, whether it's expressed mathematically or symbolically and mystically.

An alternative translation of this chant is:

> That is completely empty. This is completely empty.
> From the empty, the empty arises.
> Even when the empty is negated,
> what remains is still completely empty.

Emptiness is not a black hole (which, actually, has a ridiculous amount of mass!), but rather an open concept where there is an absence of dirt, heaviness, karmic impressions, thought waves, and thought forms that keep us mired in suffering. In the traditions of the East (including both yoga and Buddhism), emptiness is one of the most prized qualities of the spiritual aspirant. In Sanskrit, this concept is conveyed by the word *śūnyatā*. While emptiness may seem like a state that's the opposite of fullness, it is actually one and the same. Through emptying out our small concepts, thoughts, paradigms, and belief systems, we set the stage for knowing ourselves as whole, complete, and perfect.

Our limiting beliefs — which hold us somewhere between being both empty and full, in a state of suffering and uncertainty — make us constantly judge our world and ourselves, which is unnecessary and harmful to ourselves and those we judge. Casting aside judgment allows new light to be shed so we can clearly see what is in front of us and inside of us. We want to see both of these aspects. The Īśa Upaniṣad goes on to give some critically important advice to the spiritual aspirant:

> In dark night live those for whom the world without alone is real; in night darker still, for whom the world within alone is real. The first leads to a life of action, the second

to a life of meditation. But those who combine action with meditation cross the sea of death through action and enter immortality.[19]

Finding Balance: Action and Meditation

Basically, this tells us that the yogi cannot live by yoga alone. Often, when the spiritual path calls to us, it seems to call us away from our life. We find an internal landscape that had been previously ignored, and we begin to explore it through yogic pursuits such as meditation, *āsana*, and *prāṇāyāma*. Shortly thereafter, having withdrawn from our external landscape, things out there start to fall apart: relationships end, jobs are cast aside, and sometimes we even embark on a journey that removes us completely from our life and takes us to places far away and entirely out of our cultural milieu. If we don't explore this inner world, we may still envy this type of escapist excursion. But true fullness (or emptiness) cannot be brought about by escapism. Pushing away the world and life is a negation of our humanness, which is the essential vehicle for our spirit. And pushing away *anything* means that it will come back...likely with a fervor.

It's the same with our spiritual life. If we push it away, then it will haunt us from within, climbing up out of our psyche until we give it some attention and turn inward for introspection and discovery of the internal world. Both the inner and outer worlds need attention, and more importantly, acceptance. When we embrace all aspects of the inner and the outer, then we recognize the fluidity and wholeness of both. By releasing our hold on what we think our life *should* or *should not* be like, and allowing it to be what it is, then we are empty of preconceived expectations and the fullness of life can arise.

We become awesomely okay with everything.

Everything on the outside, our outer world, becomes a vehicle for exploration and realization of our habits, tendencies, patterns, and judgments — basically showing us where we are still not yet free. The darkness becomes a vehicle to reveal the light. It's the same with our inner world. Our spiritual practices reveal where we still have the tendency to overcomplicate, hold grudges against ourselves or others, or mire ourselves in small, limited thinking. It's by going to great depths that we know great heights. In the emptying out of our restrictions, we become full of potential. In this way, everything — both inner and outer — are awesomely okay. We hold the world and all its facets with acceptance and an open heart. And despite how we might be hurt, offended, or otherwise wronged, we then have the capacity to forgive, which is the ultimate expression of one who has embraced their fullness and resolved both inner and outer worlds with utter openness. In the words of Stephen Mitchell, "If you have to let go, then there was something to hold on to. When there is no offense to begin with, there is nothing to forgive.... Letting go means not only releasing the person who has wronged us, but releasing ourselves."[20]

This is how we fulfill the expression of the *pūrṇa* mantra and know ourselves to be completely whole and complete. We push away nothing, we accept everything as it is. Because it can be no other way. Acceptance allows for an enthusiastic embrace of all the parts of our life and a full participation in it. We open ourselves to possibilities that arise and ones we haven't even considered yet. We know that when things are added, we are still whole, and when things are taken away, we are still whole. We embody this elegant mantra in such a way that in the words of Śrī Brahmānanda Sarasvatī, "We are in the state where we are missing nothing": yoga.[21]

PART TWO

Traditional Kirtans

Kirtan (*kīrtana*), or the call-and-response style of chanting from the tradition of bhakti yoga, has received great popularity in our modern yoga movement. Today, we recognize the current torchbearers of this kirtan tradition, such as Krishna Das, Jai Uttal, Deva Premal, Dave Stringer, and Wah! These and many others have brought the classical Indian form of kirtan to the West and updated it for a modern, Western audience. These modern mantra musicians have revivified a practice that is said to have its roots in the *purāṇa*, where Nārada, the cosmic minstrel, chanted mantra.

Historically, we find the early roots of kirtan in the development of the bhakti yoga tradition (or the yoga of devotion). Around the ninth century or so, bardic bhakti practitioners would sing the scriptures in order to bring the stories to life, much like the way that the early Greek poets would have done. Eventually, in the sixteenth century, Caitanya Mahāprabhu (a popular leader of the bhakti yoga movement) popularized the more simplified version of kirtan chanting among the Vaishnav sect (who focus on worshiping the forms of Viṣṇu), and in particular the chanting of the Mahā Mantra (see page 153). From this point, the bhakti yoga movement became fueled by the primary practice of kirtan chanting. Kirtan arrived in the West largely through Paramahansa Yogananda (author of *Autobiography of a Yogi*), and in 1926, thousands of people packed into Carnegie Hall in New York City to chant kirtan with him. Boy, that must have been a party!

During the sixties and seventies, the hippie movement definitely helped. In particular, the Beatles' interest in kirtan gave it a popular face. George Harrison recorded a version of the Mahā Mantra in 1969, which became a hit, and of course, the Beatles sometimes included mantras in their songs (listen carefully to "Across the Universe," the mantra *jai gurudeva oṁ* is peppered throughout!). This trend has been followed by other popular musicians, including Madonna, Thievery Corporation, and Trevor Hall.

What is beautiful about the kirtan tradition is that many of the chants are not structured like some of the mantras from the Vedic texts. In fact, most are not derived from texts, but rather they were created to invoke the spirit of a particular deity. Generally, kirtan singers simply focus on the name of a deity, or even the "seed sound" (*bīja* mantra) — the vibration that houses the essence of the deity. They may chant a variety of chants to one or another aspect of the great Vedic pantheon. So while in this section you'll find specific chants to specific deities, keep in mind that largely any kirtan chant to Śiva or Kālī or Kṛṣṇa, or any aspect of them, will embody and express the same type of mythology and energy. The structure of the chant is less important than the vibration of the name invoked. The word *kīrtana* means "to cut," and the idea is that the focus on a particular name or deity helps to cut through the delusion of the mind that makes us feel separate from the source, which is being called upon, in part, by the name sung. In kirtan, the most important piece of the practice is the focus on the name, or the chosen aspect, of the chant. It is the act of calling out to that which will allow its energy and essence to arise from within, so that we know we are not separate from it, that we've "cut" through the delusion to realize we are one and the same.

As we participate in a kirtan practice, the call-and-response format generally escalates as the song progresses, culminates at a peak intensity or speed (we might additionally participate by clapping our hands or dancing), and then de-escalates and ends in a very calm, meditative way, almost like a lullaby. This reflects the arc of a spiritual practice that builds in intensity and then results in a feeling of calm and peace. At a concert, the kirtan leader will orchestrate this movement within the song, but in a yoga class, a kirtan chant may only be repeated a few times — but the essence of the arc is still there in the intention! At home, on our own, we may find that a kirtan mantra finds its way into our head and we sing it to ourselves throughout the day. We can make up the tune, say it silently, or allow it to repeat on its own within us. In this way, the repetition of the mantra can allow the energy and qualities of its chosen deity to awaken within us and shine brightly through us. No matter how we practice these mantras — alone or in a filled concert hall — they help to enliven our practice and, in turn, keep the kirtan practice alive.

And because modern-day practitioners are bringing this practice to life for us in the West, we'll find modern-day versions of chants and renderings of the music. For example, today's kirtan musicians may incorporate electric bass, synthesizers, and a full-on drum kit, in addition to the more standard classical Indian instruments like a tabla or sitar.[1] These new, popular kirtan singers have broadened the scope of the tradition so that we find kirtan music inside not only Hindu temples but also yoga studios, where teachers often include kirtan music in their playlists, or at bigger concert venues, where spiritual practitioners from a wide variety of backgrounds will gather to participate in a kirtan concert on a Saturday evening. The kirtan tradition has definitely spread through not just spiritual circles but popular circles as well.

The modern kirtan movement is a great way to immerse ourselves in traditional spiritual practices. It connects us to the roots of the tradition in a way that speaks to our Western mind-set and our American rock-and-roll hearts. Music brings our spirit to life, and as untraditional as a modern expression of kirtan may seem, it still holds the reverent thread of the great tradition it comes from. There is nothing lost in reinterpreting it for our modern cultural matrix if we hold true to the intention behind the music, which is the sacred name that carries within its vibration the potential to realign and revivify our heart and spirit.

12. Sarasvatī Invocation

Sarasvatī is the goddess of art, learning, and music. Her luminous form is clothed in pure white, and all of her adornments reflect the white purity of her spirit. She holds the power of speech, the wisdom of the Veda, and the notes of the Indian musical scale begin in her honor…Sa, Re. Indeed, she is even said to have birthed the kirtan (*kīrtana*) tradition. As the creative force behind the world, Sarasvatī's invocation is an important mantra for anyone looking for support in inspired endeavors.

ॐ ऐं सरस्वत्यै स्वाहा ।

oṁ aiṁ sarasvatyai svāhā

I invoke the name of the Devi Sarasvatī and offer all that
I have to her

Advice for Chanting

Because Sarasvatī is the goddess of art, learning, and music, this invocation is appropriate to say in the context of any learning environment. She is also the matron goddess of teachers, so a teacher could use this mantra to empower his or her teachings and allow them to both be heard and received clearly.

Sarasvatī: Goddess of Music and Sound

This mantra is said to bring the power of speech, known as *vāk siddhi,* to those who repeat it regularly. Hidden within Sarasvatī's name is the root *vāk,* which has the same root as the words *vocal, voice,* and *vox.* Her name has the power of all sound behind it, and she is the voice bestride the breath in our own body. Her vehicle is the great swan,[2] or *haṁsa,* whose name repeated over and over eventually becomes the great silent mantra of the breath: *so'ham* (see The Three Mahāvakyas, page 111). The swan is rumored to have the unique ability to separate milk from water, symbolically representing the knack for discerning what will lead toward the truth and what will lead away

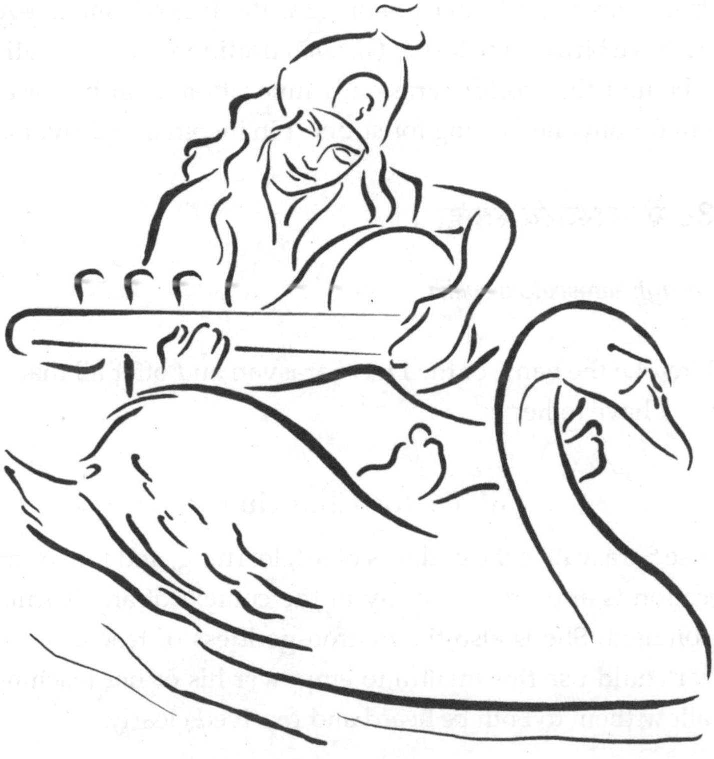

— separating the "wheat from the chaff," as we might say. This power of discernment, or *viveka,* is a key quality to cultivate along the spiritual path, as there is no "good" or "bad" in spiritual life; there is only what will lead us toward freedom and what will lead us away. Discernment is the intuitive instinct that will help us to ride the razor's edge along the road to ultimate freedom, or *kaivalya*.

The goddess Sarasvatī rides the swan of discernment, and wielding this particular vehicle gives her direction that paves the way for true knowledge — not just of the arts, literature, or scripture, but true knowledge of the highest self. Ultimately, this is where Sarasvatī is guiding us with her ever-flowing grace. Rumored to have once been a grand river that was the cradle of the Vedic civilization, Sarasvatī's life-giving waters are said to have sustained the development of the knowledge that has been passed down to us over the millennia. It is through her that knowledge is transferred by the sacred words and sounds of Sanskrit (Saṁskṛta), and it is from her that music is said to have arisen. She is seen playing the *vina,* and the sweet sounds of her playful melody have become the kirtan tradition that we know and love today.

Sarasvatī's Flowing River

Sarasvatī's flowing presence of sound, music, and wisdom are channeled into her form as a luminous lady atop her white swan and a pink lotus. Because of her unsoiled essence, and spontaneous birth from the mind of Brahmā, she was long said to be a maiden who never married or had children because the children of her spiritual wisdom were progeny enough.

Yet there is one story where she appears as one of the three wives of Viṣṇu, along with Lakṣmī and the mighty river goddess Gaṅga. Sarasvatī witnessed an intimate moment between

Gaṅga and Viṣṇu, and she became engulfed with jealousy and rage. She confronted Viṣṇu and asked him how he could be so callous and spend more time with Gaṅga than with her or Lakṣmī. He tried to explain to her that he loved them all equally, but this did not satisfy Sarasvatī. When Viṣṇu went away on business one evening, Sarasvatī picked a fight with Gaṅga, grabbing the long, flowing locks of her liquid hair, and dragged her around India, where the Ganges River flows today. Lakṣmī tried to stop the fight, and Sarasvatī cursed her and turned her into a tree for getting in the way. Sarasvatī then cursed the Ganges that she would forever carry the dead bodies and bones of the people in her waters (which she does, particularly in the Indian city of Vārāṇasi, where death rites are performed). When Viṣṇu returned home to find only Sarasvatī, he was so angry that he cursed her that her only form on earth would be that of a river, whose abundant waters would eventually dry up so that she would then only exist on the tongues of those who speak her name.

And that she does. While there is no Sarasvatī River in India today, Sarasvatī's spirit still graces the hearts and speech of those who invoke her name. As the source of all that flows and the intelligence that is constantly being expressed by the universe, Sarasvatī becomes a wellspring of inspiration and recognition of our creativity. As the goddess of sound, she is also the goddess of silence. In both science and myth, silence is the source of the creative universe, and the building blocks of the universe are sound. It seems fitting that the goddess of music would prevail over this principle and give us mythical insight into the music of the spheres, as well as the music found within our own hearts.

This is the internal nature of our own creative wellspring, our source of elevated wisdom and the internal knowledge that we are whole, perfect, and complete. To understand this is to embody it, to live it and to breathe it. And when the breath is clear, the way we convey it will uplift others merely with the sound of our voice and song, just like Sarasvatī. Her swan is our breath. Her music is our sound. Let us sing in celebration of that radiant vibrational numinosity.

13. Śrī Rām Jai Rām

The most important journey is the one we take for ourselves. Sometimes it requires us to fight the battle for our soul and slay our demons in order to realize the importance of this journey. When we're in the middle of this battle, we need a cry, one that calls out to the king or queen inside of us to inspire us on this legendary battlefield.

श्री राम् जै राम् जै जै राम् ।

śrī rām jai rām jai jai rām

Luminous King Rāma! Hail Rāma! Hail, Hail Rāma!

Advice for Chanting

Because this chant calls to our inner king (or queen), this is a great chant for when we need a little extra "oomph" or power to be brave and overcome a challenge. It is also a chant that helps to brighten up the inner light so that it can shine through any dark patterning that is holding us back and enable us to be strong in order to break through it.

Invoking Rāma and the Hero Within

This chant beckons forth the inner hero that is waiting to manifest our fullest potential, which is portrayed eloquently in the epic tale of the Rāmāyana — the story of King Rāma, Queen Sītā, and their best friend, Hanuman. We are all born kings and queens in the world who lose our love and spirit in the forest of the unconscious, and we have to reclaim it in order to find our way home.

In nearly every moment of our lives, each of us has critical choices to make, each of whose outcome inevitably determines our course in life. It is only when we walk in accord with this so-called destiny, or dharma, that the meaning and inherent value of our life unfold. The Rāmāyana is the journey of Rāma's dharma, and the course of his life reveals the power in every choice he makes.

As all great tales begin, once upon a time in a land far, far away, there was a mighty king named Daśaratha of Ayodhyā. He had four sons, the greatest of whom was known as Rāma. Rāma was beloved by his people, and when it was time for Rāma to step into his father's shoes as king, the entire kingdom rejoiced. However, the mother of his half-brother thought it was a travesty that her son, Bharatha, was not ascending to the throne. Through the power of an age-old promise made to her by Daśaratha, she then compelled Daśaratha to give the throne instead to Bharatha. Even Bharatha thought that Rāma was the better choice and tried to discourage his mother's wishes. However, the power of promises made and the sacredness of speech at this time had a binding effect, and unfortunately, what was said could not be undone. And so, against everyone's best hopes and wishes, Bharatha was crowned the new king of Ayodhyā, and his brother Rāma was banished to the forest.

As Bharatha said good-bye to his beloved brother, he vowed to keep the throne safe and to rule the kingdom wisely throughout the term of Rāma's banishment — fourteen long years. Rāma was accompanied by his fair wife, Sītā, and another loyal brother, Lakṣmana, to wander the vast forest alone. The forest contained hermits, ancient beasts, enemies, and friends. It contained mysterious caves and shape-changing creatures, and it ultimately revealed to Rāma the path to self-discovery. After fourteen years, as the brothers and beloved wife were ready to return home, the evil demon Rāvaṇa kidnapped Sītā and stole her away to his remote island of Lanka. This abduction compelled Rāma out of the forest and into his rightful place on the throne of Ayodhyā as king, where he could fight the war with Rāvaṇa to win back not only the confidence of his kingdom but the love of his beautiful wife.

While in this dark forest, Rāma encountered a great band of monkeys who were willing to help in his cause. The greatest of these monkeys, Hanuman, became his best friend. Ultimately, Hanuman's service and devotion to Rāma were of paramount importance to Rāma's ability to wage war, win the battle, and reclaim his lady wife. Without Hanuman, Rāma would have lost everything.

In the end, Rāma prevailed, as good always prevails over evil. Rāvaṇa was defeated and slain, and Sītā returned to her beloved husband. During her long captivity, her heart never wavered in her love for him. To this day, Hanuman is revered as the greatest friend and most loyal warrior and servant of the heart.

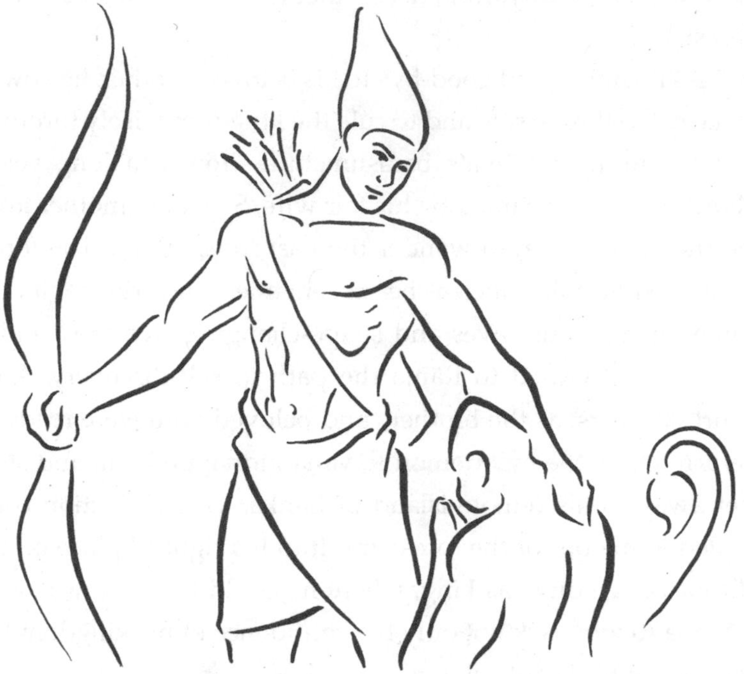

Rāma and the Hero's Journey

Great myths serve as metaphors for our own existence and as revelatory tools for our personal path. Rāma is an avatar (*avatāra*) — a prepackaged form of god who has arrived on earth to aid humanity in returning to a more elevated state based on dharma. Dharma can be defined as the cosmic order of things, the social order of things, and the personal order of things, all of which uphold one another. As he is in a human body, Rāma is inherently forgetful of his divinity, and he ends up wandering in the dark forest for fourteen years before stepping up to the plate to uphold the purpose of his existence! It makes one wonder... how, then, is a hero born?

The trajectory is simple. First, the initial push into the adventure comes. In Rāma's case, this is his apparent misfortune at losing the kingship to his brother. Often, what looks like a bummer is what starts a journey into a whole new level of awakening or heroism. But, in order to awaken, most heroes have to go through some kind of struggle to unearth their demons — both real and imagined. Rāma finds these as he enters the forest, where he wanders for fourteen years. This is a metaphorical retreat into his unconscious whereby the demons of his shadow side must be met and vanquished in order for him to leave. What happens next is the crux of the adventure, the moment when the hero of the story becomes the hero: The evil demon, Rāvaṇa, abducts Rāma's beloved Sītā. This, finally, inspires Rāma to leave the dark forest.

This story follows an archetypal trajectory, and in fact, these mystical stories are meant to serve as perfect metaphors for our own lives. King Rāma is born a god, and yet he still has to overcome the trials and tribulations of a mere mortal before finally overcoming his shadows and defeating the evil demon to allow good to prevail over evil. We often spend our early years learning about and believing in our true potential, only to wander in the metaphorical forest of unconsciousness before finally, hopefully, returning to reclaim the grandeur of this precious life. Rāma has helpers, as we have helpers. He has his family (Lakṣmana), he has his spirit (Sītā), and he has the power of his heart (Hanuman). The catalyst for his readiness to play his role, or in yogic terminology, to live his dharma, finally arises with the abduction of his spirit by evil forces.

It is in this moment that the hero decides his or her fate.

We are also heroes. When this fateful moment arises for us, we choose to either become the hero of our own story and give meaning and purpose to our own lives or remain unconscious, wandering the dark forest forever. As mystics, yogis internalize these mythic metaphors. We see how the story plays out in our own lives and conditions. This is why Joseph Campbell would encourage us to "follow our bliss." (For more on this, see the Oṁ Namaḥ Śivāya mantra, page 181.)

Following that bliss may not always be easy. It may not always be the path of least resistance. There may still be dragons or demons to slay while we're on the path, but it is what makes life worth living because it is *our* path. For Rāma, Sītā is what makes life worth living. She is his spirit — pure, untouched, perfect, and transcendent. The loss of that, of her, is staggering, as there is nothing more debilitating than an amputated soul. We see this unfortunate circumstance played out in daily life in the state of the potential hero who has either not yet heard or not yet heeded his or her own call.

Rāma's call comes loud and clear, and it is the kick start necessary to affirm his own divinity and utilize all his resources to become the king that lovers of the epic Rāmāyana story know him to be all along. His greatest asset in the ensuing fight is the representative of his heart, the glorious, faith-filled primate Hanuman. Hanuman is propelled across oceans and moves mountains solely because of his love for Rāma. At the end of the story, Hanuman rips open his chest to reveal the contents of his heart, showing benevolent onlookers images of Rāma and Sītā contained therein. In this way, Hanuman is Rāma's own heart beating outside of his chest.

And sometimes life happens that way.

Our children. Our pets. Our loved ones become external touchstones of our own individual hearts. They become those who get us through the most difficult times imaginable. It may have been impossible for Rāma to fight the battle of his life on his own. But, with Hanuman by his side, he successfully restores dharma to his dynasty. For us, as mystics, we have most certainly had personal battles that would have been quite impossible without someone we love believing in us just a little more than we believe in ourselves. When we fight our most fearsome foes, we will prevail when we are fighting with our whole heart in order to liberate our spirit. This is how we slay our own demons and dragons — whether they are found in the office, in relationships, or in addiction. We prevail when we understand the critical importance of what is at stake and what we are capable of when we have the power of love by our side.

Ultimately, Rāma wins his battle and navigates his path toward love and inspiration back in his kingly court. Rāma returns to his kingdom, and his story is sung by his two young bardic sons across time and space to reach even the most contemporary listeners. It is when one hero conquers his fear and then returns to inspire another that his tale is complete. The precious gem of the return of the hero is evidence…evidence of knowing that it is possible to become heroes ourselves. And so, the cycle continues as each of us comes to understand ourselves to be the heroes of our very own story. Like Rāma, we become kings when we stop wandering in the forest of the unconscious. Like Rāma, we become empowered when we know the value of having love on our side. And like Rāma, we know ourselves to be whole and complete when we will do whatever it takes to liberate our precious spirit and walk the path of our own hero's journey. As Joseph Campbell reminds us:

> We have not even to risk the adventure alone, for the heroes of all time have gone before us. The labyrinth is thoroughly known. We have only to follow the thread of the hero path, and where we had thought to find an abomination, we shall find a god. And where we had thought to slay another, we shall slay ourselves. Where we had thought to travel outward, we will come to the center of our own existence. And where we had thought to be alone, we will be with all the world.

14. Kālī Durge Namo Namaḥ

In greeting the goddess, or *devī*, in our kirtan, we commonly raise our voices to the aspects of Kālī and Durgā. These ladies are often seen as ferocious and feisty, when they actually embody utter compassion and kindness. Durgā, as the goddess of war, is seen riding a lion, with her ten arms holding ten different weapons. Kālī, the goddess of death, whose skin is black as night, drips blood from her mouth and wears a necklace of severed heads. Durgā and Kālī can be frightening, but they really stand before us ready to scare our fears and doubts away and invite us to integrate every part of ourselves into a unified whole. Like loving mothers who will do anything to protect their children, we find that Kālī and Durgā fight the hardest of battles in the ongoing pursuit of happiness and freedom. When we sing their names, the chant brings us closer into the fold of their skirts for protection…even if the skirt is a collection of severed arms!

जै माता काली जै माता दुर्गे ।
काली दुर्गे नमो नमः ।

jai mātā kālī jai mātā durge
kālī durge namo namaḥ

Hail mother Kālī, Hail mother Durgā,
Kālī and Durgā, we sing your name!

Advice for Chanting

A chant to Durgā and Kālī is appropriate for any situation in which we need to call upon a strong mothering force, or any time we are faced with overwhelming resistance that we hope to vanquish and reconcile. If we're in the middle of "the good fight," the energy of Durgā and Kālī can help us to win the battle.

The Ferocity of the Feminine: Kālī and Durgā

This chant honors both Kālī and Durgā together, as they often work together in their efforts to free us from the ties that bind us to suffering and fear. As we sing their names, we call forth their energy from within. In the mantra tradition, the name of something embodies the essence of its form. This is called *nāmarūpa* (meaning "name is form"). By saying the name of an aspect, we are embodying the spirit and nature of the aspect within ourselves. Given that yoga is a mystical tradition (in which everything is internalized), the intention of the chant is not to invoke Kālī or Durgā for outside help, but rather to find these ferocious forces within ourselves so that we can do the work that needs to be done to slay our inner demons and reconcile the light with the dark. This work might cause us to get our hands a little dirty.

It's what moms do.

We all have the mothering or feminine force within us — yes, even guys, too — and it is not afraid of doing the hard work. In fact, this is what the feminine is often known for. As a kid, we might remember Mom wiping off our face if we were messy eaters, or picking up after us and making our beds. Moms staunched the bleeding and put Band-Aids on our wounds. Not to mention the obvious grueling pain of childbirth. Giving birth is often a bloody affair. Life is messy. Moms clean it up.

The Battle of (Mother) Earth

Durgā has quite a name for herself in the pantheon of gods and goddesses in the Vedic tradition. She's the one called upon to fight the good fight when other forces can't seem to get the job done. If there's a demon that can't be beat, call upon Durgā.[3] If there is a universe overrun by *rākṣasa* (bad guys), summon Durgā to save the day.

In one story, a particularly evil demon starts to wreak havoc on the world. The gods try and stop him, but none are quite up to the task. So they call Durgā, who rides up regally on her lion steed, ten weapons in ten hands, ready to go to battle to save the children of earth.

Durgā stands firm and faces the demon head on. Durgā isn't afraid of bad guys. She whips out her scimitar, and with a mighty swipe lops the demon's head off. As blood spews from his neck, ten new heads grow in the original one's place, and every drop of blood that hits the ground turns into a new tiny demon. Durgā is furious. She won't stop until the demon is defeated, so she presses on, trying to kill the new little demons and still attacking the big one. But, every head she chops off grows ten more, and every drop of blood spawns a little demon. Very quickly Durgā becomes overwhelmed.

She gets frustrated first, but then she gets angry. In her anger, she stares the original demon down and furrows her brow in fury. That fury culminates in the appearance of Kālī directly out of Durgā's third eye. Kālī stands in front of Durgā, black as night and ready for blood. With her tongue hanging out, Kālī is hungry, and it turns out there's plenty for her to eat.

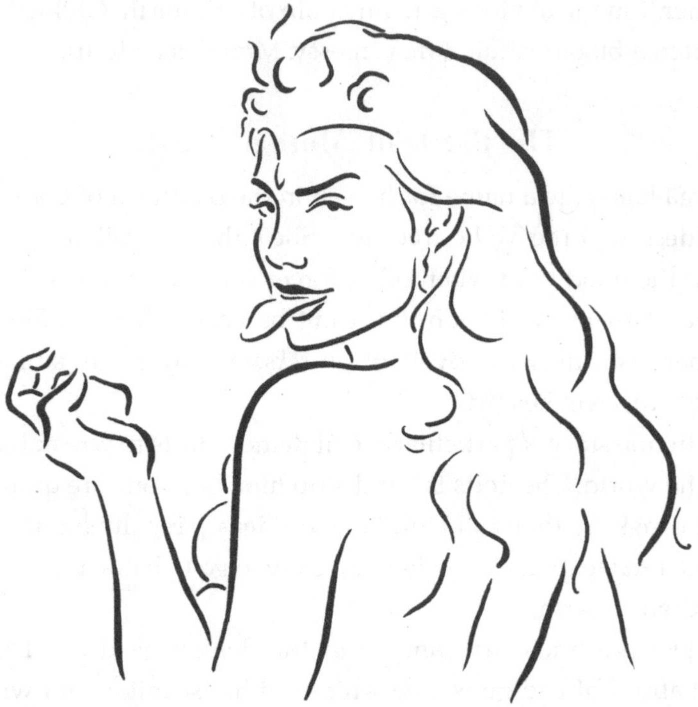

Kālī now chops off the heads of the little demons, and before any blood can hit the ground, she laps it up with her long tongue. Unable to spawn any more demons, the big demon becomes weaker and weaker as Kālī starts to make her way toward him, leaving a trail of decapitated little demons behind her. When she finally reaches the big demon, she cuts off all ten of his heads, preventing any blood from reaching the ground, and he is finally defeated and falls to the earth dead.

But Kālī isn't finished.

In her thirst for blood and knack for decapitation, she keeps going. Kālī starts to remove the heads of the forest creatures and innocent bystanders. Unstoppable and impossible to reason with, Kālī marches on in her ferocious fervor. Durgā sees this and calls an emergency meeting of the gods to try and figure out what to do with Mother Kālī. Śiva stands and holds up his right hand (*abhaya mudrā*, a symbol of fearlessness) and proclaims, "Have no fear, I know just the thing that will stop her."

Śiva incarnates on earth in a body that is completely pale white, almost ashen. He plots Kālī's path and puts himself right in harm's way, knowing that she will be upon him very soon with her hunger for death. Indeed, she is. She stomps toward Śiva as he gazes at her with a completely serene face. She pushes him down to the earth and places one foot on his chest to pin him as she is about to chop off his head. When she looks down upon him, at the moment her sword is meant to fall, she sees in his eyes perfect and unconditional love. This stops her heart and resets the beat so that she is filled with this love, too. She lowers her sword. Śiva looks at her and says, "Without you, great mother, I am dead and lifeless. With you, I am full of love and can accomplish anything."

Creating an Equal Partnership

Śiva, as a white ashen figure under the foot of Kālī, represents the masculine aspect of the universe. Kālī, in her overaccomplishing fervency, represents the feminine aspect of the universe. These two aspects must work together to strike a healthy balance that serves both their strengths and the needs of the universe. Without the feminine, symbolically, Śiva is *śava*, the corpse, lifeless underneath Kālī's foot. This lifelessness derives from too much thinking and not enough nature. Without masculine rationality and thought, Kālī, as the great feminine aspect of śakti, becomes not a giver of life but the bringer of death. Nature consumes herself like the vines in the story of Sleeping Beauty that overcome the castle while everyone sleeps inside. Shakespeare remarked on this feminine birth and death symbolism in his famous play

Romeo and Juliet when he refers to the similarities of both the womb and the tomb:

> The earth, that's nature's mother, is her tomb.
> What is her burying, grave that is her womb.

While we often think of the feminine force as being the giver and bringer of life, it is also symbolically the feminine that is the giver and bringer of death. Kālī clearly represents this apparent juxtaposition as both an aspect of the great mother and the goddess of death. Śiva is merely a static figure without the movement of Kālī. Literally, without Kālī's energy, he becomes *śava* — the corpse, embodied but immobilized without her fervent, vivifying energy. With his devotion and love to her, she is tempered enough to revivify him. They are the representation of cosmic duality, known in the yogic tradition as Śiva and Śakti. Śakti (in this case represented by Kālī) literally moves Śiva, bringing him into being and resurrecting him from his lifeless, listless state.[4]

This marriage with death brings about the true union between these pairs of opposites. Kālī, as the representative of the goddess, shows us both the "womb and the tomb" aspect of life. If we consider her as the goddess of nature and death, we can see her juxtaposition with Śiva as the god of spiritual evolution (beyond nature). Śiva's abode is high above the earth on Mount Kailāsa, practically touching the heavens, while Kālī holds dominion over the deepest part of our earthly realm and the underworld of death. When we mirror this in our psyche (as yoga's mysticism asks us to), then we see the duality of our conscious spiritual evolution and the unconscious reservoir that is hidden until we delve into it. Within the depths of our unconscious lie both the potential for the rebirth of our consciousness to even greater heights as well as the graveyard of all of our past experiences, wounds, traumas, and desires.

This duality of our consciousness and unconsciousness reflects the push-me-pull-you effect of our everyday lives, particularly when we are called to evolve to a higher state of being or a fuller expression of ourselves. We must first delve into the depths of our unconscious and bring forth what lies buried deep within us. It's as Jesus states in the Gnostic Gospel of Thomas, "If you bring forth what is within you, what you bring forth will save you. If you do not bring forth what is within you, what you do not bring forth will destroy you."[5] Spiritual evolution doesn't happen in a vacuum. We can't expect to evolve without in some way examining the nature of how we got here in the first place. We have to open up the tomb of our unconscious layers and make friends with the black figure hiding in the shadow before we can usher ourselves forth into the light to be born again as a more effulgent self.

Basically, whatever we resist on the outside is fuel for this shadow hiding on the inside underneath our conscious awareness. When we don't understand the blackness of Kālī's fervent destruction, we think she's harmful, painful, and out to get us, and she can seem out of control. Really, she shows us where we are resisting life. Like Śiva, we are *śava*, dead, without her. Our unconscious subtly rules our conscious life. All of our decisions are made by our unconscious even before our conscious mind makes them. Our unconscious governs our habits, our dreams, our nervous system, and all of our autonomic functions. Without turning a compassionate face toward the darkness, the haphazard destruction that might be buried within will continue and very important and valid parts of ourselves will remain in the tomb-like shadows.

Shadows are scary. Death is scary. Tombs are scary.

The measure of our spiritual evolution is marked by how easily we can touch the heavens while keeping our feet rooted in nature. It is when we stop resisting our shadow, when we understand its ability to reveal to us our greatest strengths, that it stops being our greatest weakness. As the representative of mother nature, both the womb and the tomb, Kālī's wrath is both fearsome and compassionate at the same time — depending on whether we walk with her into the tomb or resist it until the bitter end.

The shadow needs the light in order to reveal its depth, and the light needs the shadow in order to reveal its breadth. When we become like this image of Kālī standing on Śiva, we couple the internal aspects of light and dark and give ourselves permission to find the strength in our wounds. We feel love and openness when we are ready for Kālī to do her motherly work, to show us the shadow side and invite us into the tomb in order to reveal the life-giving nature of the power that exists within us. When we connect with that — with her, the feminine force within — then the conscious part of us, the masculine force, is brought to life, and we can manifest our whole, complete selves on the outside.

15. Oṁ Maṇi Padme Hūṁ

Of all the mantras found within the Buddhist tradition, there is one that is said to be the source of ultimate freedom, *mokṣa*, from the cycles of life and the unavoidable perils of suffering. This chant is probably much older than we know, but it was first described as a powerful mantra in a Buddhist text from about the fourth century called the Kāraṇḍavyūha Sūtra. Whether said in the mind, out loud, or written on scrolls inside great prayer wheels that allow the mantra to be said on the wind, this mantra contains the very heart of the Buddhist teachings.

ॐ मणि पद्मे हूं ।

oṁ maṇi padme hūṁ

The Jewel is in the Lotus!

Advice for Chanting

Because this mantra is said to be the greatest mantra of the Buddhist tradition, it is appropriate for anyone seeking calmness of mind and transcendence. It embodies the spirit of the boddhisattva, or one who seeks to become fully realized, like the Buddha. It will help to direct the mind toward that aim, whether said out loud or silently as part of a meditation practice.

Avalokiteśvara: Enlightenment for All

This mantra is associated with Avalokiteśvara, whose name means "The Supreme Lord who Looks Down." It's not that Avalokiteśvara is looking down on us, but rather that he is looking down upon us. This boddhisattva — as in, one who has attained Buddhahood — achieved his enlightenment and ascended to the heavenly realm, but he made a vow to stay on the earthly plane until every single being had achieved a state of *mokṣa* or nirvana. Basically, this guy agreed to keep working and teaching until every creature — man, beast, and bug — realizes the true nature of the self, which is whole, complete, and perfect. That's a lot of work.

Luckily, there's a way for us to help ourselves. Through chanting this mantra, we are recalibrated to a state where we can understand the true jewel in the lotus, which is said to be the sacred gem of true wisdom that is contained within the preciously folded lotus petals of the heart. The gleaming facets of our true nature shine outward from within to be readily accessed and understood by those who take the time to look. Avalokiteśvara did this while sitting upon a beach and meditating on the sounds of the ocean. While listening (*nāda* yoga), he heard the subtle rise and fall of the waves and realized their inseparability from the ocean. In this way, he came to the question, "What is form, and what is emptiness?" He realized, as famously said in the Buddhist Heart Sutra, that "emptiness is form and form is emptiness."[6] Emptiness, in this case, is the state that is completely without quality or fluctuation, known as *śūnyatā* (see the Oṁ Pūrṇam Adaḥ mantra, page 119).

It is within emptiness that we come to know the nature of all things as interconnected. Like the fabled net of Indra cast over all existence, every being exists at a jewel-laden juncture of the web. Each facet reflects outward from itself and shines the light of its true nature. From each juncture, as in a room of mirrors in a funhouse, sometimes it is difficult to see anything but what we are reflecting back onto ourselves. This is karma, the self-limiting cycle of madness that keeps us bound to limiting beliefs and paradigms. When we can shift our perception so the mirrors are turned outward, we then reflect the truth of our Buddha nature to everyone on the net. When this occurs, when we realize our own boddhisattva-ness, then the net is lifted a little, and that ascension pulls on all the strings of the web, taking the rest of creation with it.

So, as Avalokiteśvara works for the enlightenment of all beings, the most important thing that we can do is work toward our own spiritual elevation. By freeing ourselves from our karma, by locating the gem of our self-reflecting awareness, we become moor posts for others to attach to and be inspired by. By enlivening and enlightening ourselves, we take the whole world with us.

16. Mahā Mantra

One of the most popular mantras in today's yoga tradition is the Mahā Mantra. Made mainstream by the movement of the International Society for Krishna Consciousness (ISKCON for short), the Mahā Mantra has infiltrated into our Western spiritual psyche, not just through its notoriety within ISKCON, but in conjunction with popular musicians like the Beatles and Thievery Corporation. Originally popularized by the sixteenth-century bhakti yoga leader Caitanya Mahāprabhu, this mantra is found in a Vaishnavite (Vishnu-based) text called the Kalisantaraṇa Upaniṣad. The Mahā Mantra (literally, "great mantra") is, according to Vaishnavites and bhakti yogis, the only mantra needed for direct transcendence of the gap between highest self (*ātman*) and supreme noumenon (*paramātma*).

हरे कृष्ण हरे कृष्ण ।
कृष्ण कृष्ण हरे हरे ।
हरे रामा हरे रामा ।
रामा रामा हरे हरे ॥

hare kṛṣṇa hare kṛṣṇa
kṛṣṇa kṛṣṇa hare hare

hare rāma hare rāma
rāma rāma hare hare

Advice for Chanting

By chanting these three names, we call upon the strength of these heralded aspects of Viṣṇu:

Hare: The manifest forms of Viṣṇu, remover of delusion.
Rāma: An *avatāra* of Viṣṇu, star of the Rāmāyana, said by Vaishnavites to be an earlier embodiment of Kṛṣṇa.
Kṛṣṇa: An *avatāra* of Viṣṇu, star of the Bhagavad Gītā, considered by Vaishnavites to be the supreme form of God.

This chant is very common among devotees of the modern bhakti yoga tradition — meaning those who practice the yoga of devotion. Their primary practice is chanting, whether it be in the form of ecstatic kirtan or silent (*ajapa*) repetition of a mantra. For those who devote the focus of their energy to forms of Viṣṇu, and in particular Krishna (Kṛṣṇa), this chant can never be said enough, either out loud or silently! Feel free to use this chant any time you wish to cultivate a divine mood or internal strength. It is said to be a chant that elevates the heart to meet the heart of god.

While there are several popular ways to translate the specific words of this mantra, there is a general agreement that the great names of Viṣṇu's embodied forms (Kṛṣṇa and Rāma) are present within the chant. And though two specific *avatāra* are mentioned, this mantra specifically focuses on Kṛṣṇa and his great ability to lead hearts and minds toward the highest aim — finding balance in order to manifest our natural state of yoga.

Kṛṣṇa, Arjuna, and the Great Battle of Life

The nature of our inner, spiritual battle in life is beautifully captured in the Bhagavad Gītā, a spiritual text found within the great Indian epic the Mahābhārata. In essence, this sacred yogic text describes how the greatest warrior alive, Arjuna, fights for the restoration of righteousness with the help of only a small army and Kṛṣṇa as his chariot driver. On the eve of battle, Arjuna and his brothers play a game of dice with the leaders of the opposing army, the Kaurava brothers. The stakes of the dice game escalate, and the winners of the dice toss get to choose whether to have the more formidable army or the venerable Kṛṣṇa on their side. It's a difficult decision, but in the end, Arjuna's family wins and chooses to fight with Kṛṣṇa. The next day, Arjuna must defeat the evil Kaurava family, who have on their side an enormous army that greatly outnumbers Arjuna's piddly troops. Though it's always good to have a god on your side, Arjuna's courage falters in the moments just before battle begins.

When Arjuna rides across the battlefield to survey the opposing troops, what he sees are not faceless enemies, but rather people he knows — his distant relatives, cousins he played with as a child, the butcher and baker from down the street. These are not enemies or "others"; these are his friends, colleagues, family, and neighbors. Arjuna suddenly feels a tremendous amount of doubt about waging war against these friends, and he returns to his chariot, slumps down, and tells Kṛṣṇa, "I can't do it."

Kṛṣṇa stands tall and gives Arjuna a stern face and says, "You must fight."

"But I don't want to! I just want to run off into the forest and be a yogi. Oh, Kṛṣṇa, isn't it better to lay down my arms and walk away than to go into this battle that I'm sure to lose?" asks Arjuna. It is a good question. However, Kṛṣṇa's answer encourages Arjuna to fight, and not only to wage battle, but to make the

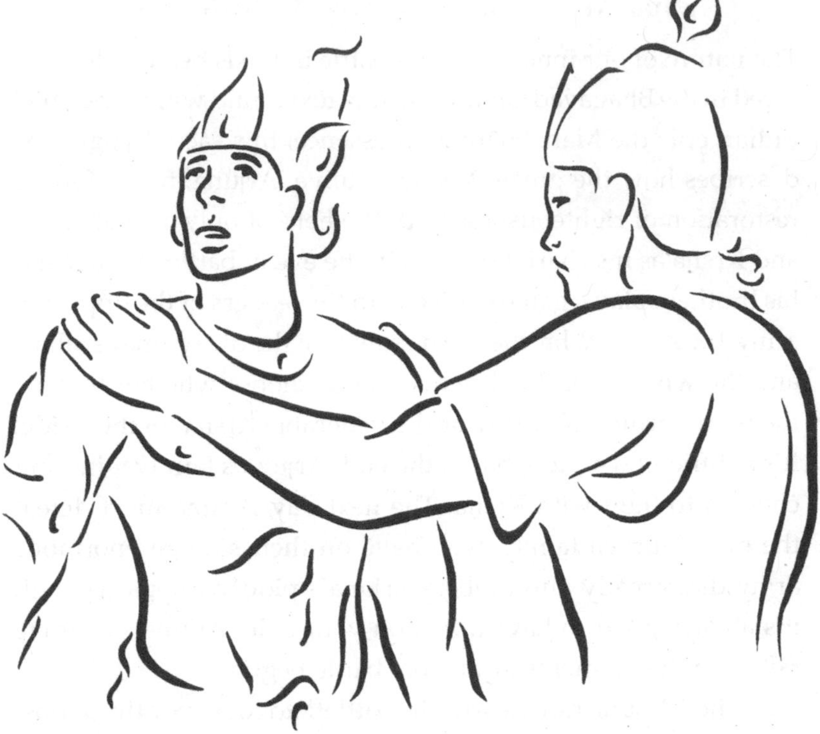

act of war his practice of yoga, for every action we take has the opportunity to free us if we can do the action in a selfless way without any attachment to the outcome.

Kṛṣṇa then counsels Arjuna about the importance of doing one's duty — of fulfilling one's dharma. Even still, Arjuna's doubt is so great that Kṛṣṇa stops time and has a dialogue with Arjuna, answering all his most important questions. This dialogue becomes the text of the Bhagavad Gītā.[7] In it, we find answers to life's most pressing questions, such as: Who am I to fight the good fight? What if I just want to give up? And a perennial favorite, Why me?

Kṛṣṇa, as an avatar of Viṣṇu and representative of supreme consciousness, explains that a yogi is one who turns his or her face toward a challenge, musters up every ounce of courage available, and draws the tools necessary for the fight. Only by engaging in the fight, even if it comes unasked to our doorstep, can we achieve balance in the world. Balance is part of the complex notion of dharma. While dharma means one's "duty" in an everyday sense, it also refers to the duty we each have to uphold the integrity of our lives, which then reflects as balance and integrity in the world. This spiritual duty is paramount, and pursing or defending it is not easy. It results in casualties. Like the conflict facing Arjuna, the battle ahead is long, and many will die. But Kṛṣṇa reminds Arjuna that he is merely acting out his earthly duty as part of the divine cosmic play. In this way, Kṛṣṇa makes clear that our challenges in life are always only representations of the inner struggle to achieve spiritual balance.

Life's Toughest Challenge: Becoming the Spiritual Warrior

Naturally, after Kṛṣṇa's pep talk, Arjuna kicks ass and wins that day. But it still isn't easy. Living ain't easy. As this story makes clear, life isn't always about sparkles, rainbows, and butterflies. Life is stuffed with a myriad of challenges, but the central one is the mere fact of being human. And though humans have limitations — we are imperfect; we have egos, fears, and desires — we also have a brilliant spark within us that will always light the way. This is illustrated in the Bhagavad Gītā with the juxtaposition of the roles of Arjuna and Kṛṣṇa.

The brilliance of the mythology of the Bhagavad Gītā is that it presents so clearly a template for our everyday condition. Remember, yoga is a mystical practice that regards everything from an internalized perspective. So Arjuna's story is not about a warrior fighting an actual battle, but a metaphor for our own inner champion, our own warrior, who is ready to stand and fight the good fight, even when the going gets tough. And it's precisely when the going gets tough that Viṣṇu appears, in the guise of one embodied form or another, and reminds us that each battle is an opportunity for us to move deeper into our spiritual center. Our duty, our dharma, is to put aside ego and connect to the numinous and the world around us.

Further, at heart, despite all his doubt, Arjuna knows he is not alone. He knows Kṛṣṇa has his back. In this way, we also know that in the darkest moments of our lives, there is a higher part of us that draws from vast wisdom and a deeper place within ourselves. When we access this, we can manifest our greatest potential and lift ourselves up to meet all of the greatest challenges we face with courage, inner strength, and fortitude. For Arjuna's real battle isn't the one he fights on the battlefield, it's the one he fights with himself to know that he is capable of winning the war. Indeed, he's the only one that is. Knowing this, and following through in the spirit of selflessness is what makes him a yogi — the great spiritual warrior.

17. Gaṁ Gaṇapataye Namaḥ

One of the most popular of all the deities in the yogic pantheon is Gaṇeśa (Ganesh), who inspires loyalty through his charming presence and generous ability to help out with problems, though usually in a clever way that we might not expect. Gaṇeśa's helpful and lively qualities are well renowned — he is known for his great balance as he rides a mouse, despite his heft and elephant head. He is also recognized as a regular yoga practitioner, which he learned from his father, Śiva, the founding father of yoga. Gaṇeśa is also a great listener, given his large elephant ears. He is happy to listen to the troubles of those who call upon him in order to help find a crafty solution. The simple kirtan chant presented here combines the seed sound for Gaṇeśa, *gaṁ* — which harnesses the very essence of his uncanny problem-solving abilities — with a call for refuge in Gaṇeśa's delightful energy.

गं गं गं गणपतये नमः ।
गणेष शरणं गनेश शरणं ।
शरणं गणेश शरणं गणेश ॥

gaṁ gaṁ gaṁ gaṇapataye namaḥ
gaṇeśa śaraṇaṁ gaṇeśa śaraṇaṁ
śaraṇaṁ gaṇeśa śaraṇaṁ gaṇeśa

Gaṁ, gaṁ, gaṁ, I call the name of sweet Gaṇapati
I seek refuge in Gaṇeśa's protection

Advice for Chanting

Gaṁ is Gaṇeśa's seed sound, or *bīja* mantra, which contains the essential energy of Gaṇeśa (as all *bīja* mantras do). A *bīja* mantra is like the seed of the banyan tree that carries within it all the potential for the great tree itself. Seed sounds, which can express the seed of a deity, a chakra, or energy — or even the universe, as *oṁ* does! — provide the core vibration that blooms fully into the expression they reference. *Gaṁ* is the little seed that houses the vibration of everything about Gaṇeśa. Just like the universe (see the Asato Mā mantra, page 47), every good idea begins with a seed. This mantra allows us to plant seeds for the solutions to our problems. Gaṇeśa's essential energy helps us with this, and so we can use this chant any time we feel a blockage and are seeking a solution.

This mantra has pieces that we can use separately or together. It is fine to simply chant the *bīja* mantra on its own, silently or out loud, in order to plant quick, effective, problem-solving seeds. The second part of the chant — *gaṇeśa śaraṇaṁ* — can also be used on its own if the feeling you are looking to cultivate is some protection from the problem at hand. The word *śaraṇaṁ* means "refuge," the idea being that we can take shelter in the ensuing storm and ride it out until the light comes. Of course, as yogis, we are looking for the protective light of our own wisdom that has a higher perspective on the storm. We're looking for the aspect of Gaṇeśa within us to protect us from the stormy mental onslaught that sometimes occurs while obsessing over a problem.

Gaṇeśa: Remover of Obstacles

Gaṇeśa is hailed as the remover of obstacles, and so he has garnered popularity for his ability to make all things go smoothly. However, Gaṇeśa's real power lies not in his physical strength but in his intelligence. He reveals unexpected resolutions to every challenge or sees challenges in ways that transform them into possibilities. In other words, Gaṇeśa doesn't blast away the rock that blocks our path, but he shows us the way around the rock, how to tunnel underneath it, or how to see the rock as the destination our path was meant to lead to. Gaṇeśa's real power is his ability to create a shift in perception. By shifting our perception, we see that every problem has an inherent resolution. Often, in fact, the solution is this shift in perception, as we realize the problem was only a problem because of the way we viewed it. Gaṇeśa is not the remover of obstacles, but rather, the revealer of possibilities.

The refuge that the chant invokes with the Sanskrit word *śaraṇaṁ* is similar to the feeling we get when we are snuggled up in a cozy blanket in a safe place. When we take refuge within a particular energy, we surrender ourselves to it and allow it to saturate us from the outside in. This is particularly appropriate with Gaṇeśa, for his outlook on life is essentially that there are no problems. Basically, he's awesomely okay with everything, including himself. He radiates a calm gaze and sharp focus. Problems do not bother him because he does not resist them or try to avoid them or out-muscle them. Rather, he accepts them and adjusts his attitude and perspective to meet them, and so he reveals the intrinsic power "problems" hold for us.

The following mythic story captures not only Gaṇeśa's genius, but his ability to find a clever solution to a problem. As the son of Śiva and Pārvatī, Gaṇeśa's royal birth set him high in the ranks of the gods. His brother, Skanda, often took advantage of their popularity and developed a bit of an attitude, thinking himself far cooler than some of the other gods.

One day, Śiva and Pārvatī witness this behavior and decide to stir things up a bit. They devise a test between Gaṇeśa and Skanda to determine which of the boys will be the "favorite" and garner the most accolades and acknowledgment, not just from them, but from the world.

Śiva and Pārvatī bring the boys together and inform them of the test. Skanda is immediately sure he will win, even before he learns the nature of the test itself. Gaṇeśa stands coolly by, waiting for his father to explain. Śiva places his arm around Pārvatī and says, "Okay, whichever of you boys can circumnavigate the universe three times the fastest and return here first will win our grandest favor forever."

With that, Skanda races off.

Already known as the fastest of the gods, he can't believe that his parents have created a test between him and his brother that he is so sure to win! There is no chance that Gaṇeśa, with his fat body and big elephant head, will ever be able to beat him in a race. And, as Skanda rounds his first turn of the universe and passes his family, he sees that Gaṇeśa is still standing there.

"What is he thinking? He must have just given up!" thinks Skanda.

Skanda doesn't even lose his breath as he rounds the universe a second time. When he runs past his family, he catches a glimpse of Gaṇeśa and sees a little twinkle in his eyes. He tries not to let it faze him as he continues his third turn around the universe.

Just then, Gaṇeśa starts to shuffle coolly and calmly around his parents, circling Śiva and Pārvatī once…twice…and three times, before finally standing beside them both with his arms around their shoulders.

Just then, Skanda races up behind them and shouts, "I did it! I won! I'm the favorite!"

"No, I'm sorry, son, but you've lost," says Śiva.

"What? How is that possible?" Skanda replies in exasperation. He'd been so fast! Gaṇeśa never passed him; in fact, he'd never even seen Gaṇeśa move from the starting line. This must be some mistake or cruel joke.

Śiva then explains that Gaṇeśa circled him and Pārvatī three times. As the ultimate sources of the universe, Gaṇeśa had simply gone around his parents, as opposed to circumnavigating their outer expression, all of creation. Skanda had missed the big picture and lost sight of the forest for the trees, so to speak. Gaṇeśa had found the simplest answer, and in so doing, he solved the challenge with the least amount of effort.

Problems Are in the Eye of the Beholder

Gaṇeśa, in his simplistic and elegant wisdom, traces each challenge to its source. He sees problems as not being "out there" but as being right in front of him, or we might say, as part of him. He knows that since his parents are the source of the universe, all he needs to do is embrace them to have the whole thing encircled. There is no racing, no striving, no running or straining involved. The simplest, most localized act solves the task.

When faced with a problem, we needn't look outside of ourselves, whether to blame others, or to offload the problem, or to find someone to fix the problem for us. Gaṇeśa's wisdom points us within, where the source of each problem lies. Whatever the problem is, it doesn't matter. The simple fact that we view it as a problem is what makes it a problem.

For example, one person's problem is often another person's

spiritual challenge, great opportunity, or rite of passage. The way we view a situation is what makes it what it is, and our attachment to our perspective is usually the real problem. This idea is captured by a well-known Eastern parable.

One day, a man decides to play the lottery, and he wins. His neighbors all congratulate him on his good fortune.

He responds with, "Good? Bad? We'll see!"

The neighbors think he is a little funny, but they watch all the same as the man uses his winnings to build a new house. He moves into his house with his wife. During a freak storm, the new house falls on his wife, injuring her. The neighbors all come to offer their sympathies for the man's misfortune.

He responds with, "Good? Bad? We'll see!"

While the man visits the hospital, he notices that his wife also has another visitor. Another man. Apparently she's been having an affair. The neighbors find out and congratulate the man on revealing the infidelity of his wife.

He responds with, "Good? Bad? We'll see!"

The man goes home and starts to fix his house. But it costs him all the remaining money he won in the lottery. The man is once again broke. The neighbors sadly come to see the man off as he sells his house and moves out.

He responds with, "Good? Bad? We'll see!"

As the man leaves his house, he runs into an old high school crush. They get to talking. He tells her all he's been through. He shares the events and waits for her reaction.

She responds with, "Good? Bad? We'll see!"

They continue walking down the road together.

In other words, all challenges contain blessings and all blessings contain challenges. Our work, like the work of Gaṇeśa, is not to get caught up in whatever arises, but rather to see what each situation reveals to us about ourselves. When an obstacle appears, and we resist it, we then see exactly where we are not free. If the problem is financial, we see our own limiting beliefs around money. If the problem is physical, our limiting beliefs about our body are revealed. If the problem is in our relationships, then we see our limiting beliefs around who we are in relationships and how relationships are supposed to go. This is particularly valuable information.

On the spiritual path, we are interested in freedom from limiting beliefs. Limits are like prison walls keeping us from manifesting our greatest potential. If we stay behind those bars, we've got nothing but problems all the time. When we free ourselves from these bonds, then we are free to roam wherever we like. Just as Gaṇeśa maneuvered coolly around his parents, we can maneuver coolly around our lives when we learn to shift our perceptions in ways that reveal not problems, but possibilities.

18. Jai Ambe Jagad Ambe

This chant is a general chant to the goddess, the all-encompassing mother force that is manifested through different incarnations. Whether it be the various goddesses of the Eastern traditions, the Mother Mary, or our own mother — this chant invokes the mother (*mātā*) of the world (*jagad*). Of course, in the internal, mystical reading of this chant, we focus our energy on anything within us that nurtures, supports, or "births," whether we are giving birth to an idea, a business, or a baby! When we want to bring forth this powerful generative and supportive force within us, or if we want to honor the feminine in her life-giving aspect, we can use this chant.

जै अम्बे जगद् अमबे ।
माता भवानि जै अमबे ॥

jai ambe jagad ambe
mātā bhavani jai ambe

Hey mother, mother of the world,
The mother who gives, we honor you.

Advice for Chanting

We hear this chant often in a kirtan setting, and it can be easily done as a call-and-response chant. Another way in which this chant might be used is in a *pūjā*, which is a ritual-type ceremony that honors a particular aspect and invokes that aspect's energy. It is very common in India and in the yogic tradition to start the day with a small, personal *pūjā*. An altar can be built with one's favorite, most sacred items and an image of the chosen aspect or deity. Then, chanting is done to honor that deity and increase the sacrality of the altar itself. This also becomes like a prayer that asks for that aspect to come through strongly in one's life. While one could choose any deity and its associated chants, this chant will be particularly effective in bringing forth a nurturing energy in one's life. Specifically, one could focus the energy of this chant on the popular goddess of abundance, Lakṣmī (Lakshmi), in order to create more abundance of all kinds in one's life.

Lakṣmī, the Goddess of Fortune and Abundance

The world, Mother Nature, our planet. All these names reflect various titles of the great feminine goddess that cultures across time have recognized as the source of life. It is from her that we arise, and it is back to her that we go. The ancient Greeks had Gaia, South American peoples have Pachamama, the Christian tradition has Mother Mary, and in the East, the goddess has many names. They are each thought to be aspects of the great mother from whom all life is given.

Many of us are familiar with the mother's life-giving aspect and her multifaceted ability to get things done. In fact, without the feminine power of śakti, the masculine forms are lifeless (for more on this, see the Kālī Durge Namo Namaḥ mantra, page 141). For every masculine deity, there is a feminine goddess that fuels his power and provides his energy. Śiva has Śakti in her many forms. Brahmā has Sarasvatī (whom Brahmā brought into being from his pure thoughts). Viṣṇu has Lakṣmī. And Lakṣmī (like all mothers) has a big job! Viṣṇu, as the preserving force of the universe, needs the energy of the goddess Lakṣmī to provide abundance and grace for his precious world. Born of the churning of the oceans,[8] Lakṣmī was given the opportunity to choose her counterpart. Because Viṣṇu lies cool as a cucumber on a serpent couch, not reaching or grabbing for anything, she chose him. She enlivens his dreams and helps to bring about beauty and fortune in his universe. She is the heart of Viṣṇu, and as such, incarnates with him in each of his *avatāra* aspects. She appears as Rukmiṇī, the wife of Kṛṣṇa, and as Sītā, the lover of Rāma.

Lakṣmī is one of the most favored goddesses because she is the goddess of fortune and abundance — and so she embodies perfectly the energy and essence of this mantra. But more than just gold coins flow from her hand. As an aspect of the mother of the world, she bestows softness and radiance on the landscape, which would otherwise be flat and unmoving. Also known as Śrī, meaning "luminous," she gives us solace and, like the quintessential mother goddess, provides us with exactly what we need.

Abundance, Redefined

The well-loved goddess of abundance, Lakṣmī is a favorite because of her perceived ability to offer prosperity in times of lack. It is far more than money and riches that she offers to those who spend time invoking her energy. This is made clear in an Indian parable about one particular family who dedicated their in-home shrine to Lakṣmī. For many generations, the family offered *pūjā* (ritual worship) to her daily. This constant invocation of the goddess Lakṣmī ensured her presence in their home, and the family grew stronger and more abundant over time. Eventually, the family had two sons, one who married and one who helped to run the factory.

Then one evening, after the father's ritual *pūjā,* Lakṣmī appears to him in her full glorious form, standing on a lotus, coins in one hand, the other held up as a gesture of protection and good faith.

"My friend," she says, "I have been with your family for many generations because of your loyal reverence to me. It is time now that I leave you and spread good fortune elsewhere. But since you have been so kind and loving toward me, before I go, I will offer you one boon. Ask for anything you like, and it shall be yours."

Thinking quickly, the father turns to beautiful Lakṣmī and says, "You know, I'd like one day to think it over before I give you my answer. Please come back tomorrow."

Lakṣmī agrees and disappears, and the father goes to seek the counsel of his family. It is the family's tradition to honor Lakṣmī, so he wants the entire family involved in the decision. The man asks his wife what she would want from Lakṣmī, and she says it would be nice to have a bigger kitchen to cook bigger meals for her big family. He goes to his youngest son and asks him what he thinks Lakṣmī should bestow. The youngest son says, "We should ask her for another factory. We're doing well now, but with one more factory, we'd really be all set."

The father asks his older son, who replies, "Let's ask Lakṣmī for a big family car. That way we can drive where we want and take cross-country trips."

The father considers all these ideas and starts to think about what he'd like. What types of abundance would most benefit his family? More money? More frequent flyer miles? Perpetually full cupboards? A bigger house? Feeling overwhelmed by the decision, the father remembers his daughter-in-law and thinks, "Well, she's part of the family, too. I should ask her what she thinks!"

The daughter-in-law is in the family compound. After listening to her father-in-law explain the situation, she sits thoughtfully for a minute, then replies, "I think we should ask Lakṣmī to give us the peace of mind that we have right now. Right now, we are happy. We have everything we need. We know we are provided for, and we don't lack anything."

The father likes this idea very much. When Lakṣmī returns the next evening, she appears graceful and radiant. Looking upon him with smiling eyes, she says, "Are you ready to ask for your boon, sir?"

He nods his head and speaks confidently: "Dear Lakṣmī, I have consulted my whole family and considered many options. In the end, I have decided to ask you to always provide us with the peace of mind we have right now. Through your grace, we always feel abundant and happy with what we have. We recognize that we don't need anything more, and so we never feel lack. No matter how much or how little we have, we are always confident and at peace, knowing you will provide exactly what we need."

Lakṣmī smiles, and then laughs. "You have tricked me, clever sir! Now, I cannot leave your household because you have asked me for the one thing that I truly do provide to those who invoke my presence. Abundance comes not from coins or material items, but from the peace of mind in recognizing that you are always provided for."

Lakṣmī then returns to her place upon the family's altar, where she remains today, blessing the family with the peace of mind they asked for.

Mother Knows Best

Lakṣmī's great lesson teaches us that we always have everything we need. We often focus on what we think we lack or on what others have that we want. But in reality, we always have exactly enough. How can we know that? Because when we look back over our lives, we see that in every instance, we have had exactly what we needed to get through every situation. No more, no less. Was it hard? Sure. Could having a little more resources or knowledge perhaps have made it easier? Sure…but would we have learned the lessons necessary without a bit of struggle? Maybe not. Struggle actually helps us grow. Lakṣmī represents the peace of mind that comes when we recognize and trust that we already possess everything we need to cope with the inevitable struggles of life and so learn to thrive in all circumstances.

Even Lakṣmī, the goddess of abundance, knows that lasting abundance does not come from counting how much we have and continually adding more. It comes when we appreciate what we already possess and don't feel a need to ask for more. That's her little trick. She offers us peace of mind, no matter what our circumstances, when we recognize the self-evident abundance all around us that already exists. This is true particularly in challenging times, when grace comes through recognizing the value of our struggle.

For all the goddesses, providing the substrate for the growth and abundance of their children is paramount. Mother Earth nourishes all beings on the planet. The feminine is present in all the moments of our lives, supporting us in all of our adventures, providing us with the tools we need as well as with the peace of mind to know we're being taken care of. With this in mind, we can enthusiastically say "yes" to all the moments of our life, knowing that through the grace of the feminine, we always have enough.

19. Govinda Jaya Jaya

The most revered and loved aspect of the bhakti yoga tradition is the *avatāra* of Viṣṇu known as Kṛṣṇa. We have many stories of Kṛṣṇa's life from the texts dedicated to him, including the Śrīmat Bhagavat (also known as the Bhagavat Purāṇa) and the Bhagavad Gītā, which is a part of the larger epic the Mahābhārata. Vaishnavites and the bhakti tradition have elevated Kṛṣṇa to the highest status among the gods and also given prominence to his young love affair with the cowgirl (*gopi*) Rādhā. Here is one kirtan chant that brings their ecstatic romance to life.

गोविन्द जय जय ।
गोपल जय जय ।
राधा रमण हरि ।
गविन्द जय जय ॥

govinda jaya jaya
gopala jaya jaya
rādhā ramaṇa hari
govinda jaya jaya

Hail Hail Govinda,
Hail Hail Gopala,
In the name of Queen Rādhā,
Hail Vishnu's avatar, Govinda.

Advice for Chanting

The lively and ecstatic nature of this chant lends itself very well to the kirtan setting, which will increase the speed and vivacity of the chant, just as lovers increasingly yearn for each other. If alone, perhaps chant this line by line in a call-and-response fashion, which is a great way to learn the words and imbibe the feeling imparted by the mantra. Essentially, this chant embodies the yearning of the lover for the beloved, one who seems ever-elusive and just out of one's grasp...which seems to make the other even more desirable. As a way to develop and sustain a love for god, or one's highest self, this particular mantra will serve well.

Bhakti Yoga: The Pursuit of Devotion

Both Govinda and Gopala are affectionate names for Kṛṣṇa during his younger years as a cowherd. They mean "cow-herder" and "cow-protector." Interestingly, the prefix "go-" also alludes to the mind, and so these names additionally indicate a corralling and protecting of the mind. Very handy, particularly when the mind tends to wander! As for Govinda, his mind is focused on one thing: his main squeeze, Rādhā. Rādhā and Kṛṣṇa share an extraordinary love that the bhakti tradition sings about constantly, as it embodies the spirit of the *bhakta* — devotion.

This mantra alludes to both Govinda and his beautiful cowgirl love interest, Rādhā, as they pursue each other around the forested hills of Vṛndāvana (Vrindavan). Though Govinda continuously escapes Rādhā's grasp, she calls out from her heart to have him stand still, if even for just a moment. Then the moment shifts, and the lovely Rādhā becomes the pursued. Govinda turns toward her and follows her around the hills. Though each loves the other deeply, their love is complicated. They barely spend any actual time with each other — maybe a fleeting moment here, or a few wee hours of the morning there. Their love is never consummated by the fires of marriage. It always remains in this early romantic stage, where each is perpetually consumed by the other, in thought, word, and action.

It is this sweet separation of lover and beloved that is cultivated in the tradition known as bhakti yoga. A *bhakta*, or those who practice bhakti, call out to this sweet separation between themselves and the numinous through kirtan chanting. This continued play, known as *līlā*, is the enticing call of each beckoner to constantly seek and strive for the divine. As humans, we sometimes find it difficult to know ourselves as heavenly, holy, or wholly divine. In this forgetful state, bhakti yoga, or this devotion-filled pursuit, can be very helpful in enlivening the world around us as potential hiding places for that which we seek.

The divine play (*līlā*) between Kṛṣṇa and Rādhā is very playful. Like a great game of cat and mouse, the anticipation is what makes the game exciting, not the conclusion. Remember playing hide-and-go-seek as a child? Our heart thumps and our breath catches as we lay in wait... but, as soon as we are found, the thrill dissipates. We may even feel let down, as if we should have hid better, in some more obscure cabinet, because the chase is really what the game is all about!

This play of the bhakti yogis is all about the chase. It's about cultivating the sweetness of separation between lover and beloved, pursuer and pursued. Actually, it's a bit like dating.

Dating God

In a new relationship, everything feels alive, heightened. We become more aware of how we look, how we behave, and how we present ourselves. We'll check our smartphones twice as often to see if our love interest has texted or left a voice mail. If he or she hasn't, we double-check: is our phone service working? We spend all our free time imagining what a life with them would be like. Does he cook? Is she a morning person? What toothpaste does he use? Does she like to travel? We invent entire conversations and whole futures in our head.

As we enter into a new relationship, our whole world brightens. The colors become richer. Every compliment feels like a blessing. We are reminded of him or her in everything we touch, taste, smell, and experience. Our newly beloved is infused within our existence like a tender balm over the vulnerability of our hearts. We are soothed by the mere thought of his look, her touch, his smell, her tender caress. In this consumed state, just as in the devoted pursuit of the divine *līlā* between Kṛṣṇa and Rādhā, normal life becomes a near impossibility. We are said to be lovesick. We sign emails with little heart emoticons. Forget about paying attention to the mundanity of life. Everything pales in comparison to the shiny newness of this budding love.

And so it is with our spiritual practice, particularly with any new practices we start in order to develop a closer relationship with the sacred, or to feel that divine source more immediately in our lives. No matter what name we call the divine, this relationship becomes like a new love interest, and indeed, it is like we are dating God. That may sound irreverent, but the symptoms are the same. For instance, when people begin a dedicated yoga practice, or start a new class or technique, it often begins with a fervor. It's all we talk about. We schedule our lives around our new favorite teacher. We save all our extra pennies for yoga retreats or intensives. We recruit our friends and family to try the practice, convinced they'll love it as much as we do. We craft our wardrobe around yoga pants and slip-on shoes, wondering if yoga will think these pants look good on us. We consider our budding spirituality at every turn, always asking: "What would a yogi do?"

Basically, we are dating our spiritual practice.

Like a burgeoning relationship, we are cultivating the sweetness of the pursuit, looking for salvation around every corner. We call out to the beloved, just as Kṛṣṇa and Rādhā call to each other, just as a bhakti yogi chants the divine's name at every opportunity. But here's the catch.

Rādhā never catches Kṛṣṇa.

This is like forever "dating" someone you're completely crazy about. And yet, that's the challenge of a spiritual practice. Can we maintain that freshness and fervency through all the long years of our spiritual discipline? In his book *Outliers*, Malcolm Gladwell presents the theory that it takes ten thousand hours of practice to master any discipline.[9] If we are to achieve mastery in yoga, which is the state of complete self-confidence, self-awareness, and independence, then we must find a way to maintain our excitement and devotion to our practice, in essence, indefinitely. If we get tired or frustrated after a few unrequited turns around the tree, we'll never make it. We must take the devotion to our spiritual practice to the nth degree, particularly when the going gets tough. And it will.

No relationship is perfect or static. To stand the test of time, relationships must embrace their imperfections and evolve. In fact, Kṛṣṇa and Rādhā's relationship has its challenges — despite their love, they eventually both marry other people. In Kṛṣṇa's case, thousands of others! What they represent, then, is not some idealized romance. Rather, they represent the steadfastness of our desire to experience the divine. They embody the unquenchable devotion that persists even when what we most want remains elusive, just beyond our grasp.

By dedicating ourselves to a steady and consistent practice, we will find the strength and confidence to move through the inevitable challenges along our spiritual journey with relative grace. We will keep our eyes on the prize, as it were. If we are haphazard or inconsistent in our practice, doubts will creep up on us, the ground beneath our feet will quickly become shaky, and at the first sign of trouble, we may run the other way. We may keep seeking, hoping to find a different beloved who is easier to catch, or perhaps we will give up even trying. Our dedication — in this case, to the constant repetition of the precious mantra of our yoga practice — will be the thread we hold on to that pulls us through when we face our greatest challenges.

When we continue to deepen our relationship to our spiritual practice, we find that we are more openhearted and spacious inside, which translates to friendlier interactions and less conflict on the outside. Our practice becomes the touchstone for our human experience, a compass rose upon which to navigate.

In other words, the practice and practitioner become one and the same. Our practice vivifies us from within. Any consistently repeated spiritual practice will do this. With a mantra practice, what many find is that, eventually and sometimes after a long time, the mantra begins to chant us. We are moved by the power of these sacred practices within our lives, and eventually it is an inextricable part of ourselves. Calling to our beloved becomes the same as catching the beloved, and from this point, there is no return.

Seeing the World in Love

Indeed, at this point, you might say that one's spiritual practice less resembles a romance than partners who have been married for many decades and who have taken on the mannerisms, qualities, and even appearance of the other. In a similar way, we take on the qualities of our practice, which enlivens and shapes us from the inside out. We find this profound truth explained in the Yoga Sūtra (1.23):

> ईश्वर प्रनिधानाद्वा ।
> *īśvara praṇidhānād vā*
> Offer everything you are up to the source of your being.

While this *sūtra* instructs us to make everything we do an offering, it is how this directive works that reveals the magic of this devotional type of practice, which is at the core of bhakti, or the embodiment of devotional love. As Kṛṣṇa and Rādhā continuously devote their actions and prayers to each other, they begin to see each other in everything and all around them. The simple flower becomes a reminder of Rādhā's beauty. The song of the bird evokes the melody of Kṛṣṇa's flute. When our attention is consistently offered to the beloved, then the beloved appears everywhere and in all things. From an internal or mystical perspective, through a consistent, long-term spiritual practice, the qualities of our practice begin to appear in us and everywhere in our world. They are being projected from our center, which is in love with and devoted to the whole world.

This happens as we dedicate all of our intention and attention to our practice. The practice of mantra embodies harmony. The practices of yoga embody wholeness. Through our devotion to these practices, then, we come to experience harmony and wholeness; these qualities become who we are. Conversely, if we devote ourselves to the problems of our life, our life becomes problematic. If we devote ourselves to all that we seem to be missing, then we find what is lacking and always feel we are missing out.

And if, like Kṛṣṇa and Rādhā, we devote ourselves to the source of everlasting love, then we will come to embody love everlasting.

20. Oṁ Namaḥ Śivāya

There are many chants to Śiva, and there are many aspects of Śiva, as we have already seen in the Oṁ Tryambakaṁ mantra (page 103) and the Guru Mantra (page 33). Those mantras capture Śiva's well-known association with death. In this mantra, Śiva is presented in his highest and most all-encompassing form. This grand form of Śiva appeared originally within the Veda and then reappeared in the Śiva Purāṇa and other texts of the Shaivite tradition. The term *Shaivite* refers to those who view Śiva and his various forms as the supreme deity above all others, whereas Vaishnavites regard Viṣṇu and his various forms as the supreme deity. Shaivites believe that Śiva is not only embodied in ways that make him more personal, but that Śiva is the ultimate form of the supreme source — an impersonal form that is the essence of all things and responsible for all of creation. Śiva's all-pervading essence is said to be rooted in this great mantra:

ॐ नमः शिवाय ।
oṁ namaḥ śivāya
oṁ I invoke the supreme essence of Śiva!

Advice for Chanting

This mantra's five syllables are counted as: *namaḥ śivāya*. This mantra is said to be untranslatable because of its timelessness; this is a reference to Śiva as the ultimate, all-pervasive form of the source as well as the fact that the sounds of the syllables themselves are endless and contain great power. Each syllable is inexhaustible — there are no hard linguistic stops, and the sounds only need interrupting because we run out of breath — and each syllable is said to encompass the scope of every known aspect of the universe. When chanting this mantra, you'll often hear the *oṁ* at the beginning, which is the *bīja* mantra, or seed sound, of the universe, and so in a way, it "kicks off" the rest of these syllables. However, sometimes the *oṁ* is left off to focus only on the five syllables contained in this precious mantra. While Śiva is specifically named (*namaḥ*), the energy of this chant invokes not a specific form of Śiva, but rather his greatest form as the cosmic source, or internally, as our highest self. Chanting this mantra (either in a kirtan setting or alone) brings a clarity of mind and a sense of elevated purpose to one's life.

Śiva, the Supreme Deity

As one of the most historic gods from the Vedic tradition (and probably even before!), Śiva has a long past that has given him a variety of epithets, aspects, and incantations. Among his many names are Hara (remover of death), Rudra (remover of pain), and Maheśvara (great lord); we also understand him as the impetuous, ash-covered yogi and the lord of immortality. Originally, the name Śiva may have only been an indicator for the numinous source, or the highest self. Eventually, Śiva's various forms became more distinguished and notorious, and he developed into one of the great triumvirate alongside Brahmā and Viṣṇu. Long misunderstood as the "god of destruction," Śiva gets a bad rap that doesn't really cover the gamut of what he is capable of in this grander, more historic form. For example, Śiva's early form absorbed both Brahmā and Viṣṇu, so that he contained all three essential powers — birth, life, and death. In the Shaivite tradition, which is still very much active, devotees look upon Śiva as the god above all others and containing all others. We find this cosmic description of Śiva, known as Rudra, in the Kaivalya Upaniṣad:

> He is the Creator, the lord of sleep,
> And Indra, the lord of heaven;
> Indestructible, supreme, self-resplendent.
> He is the Pervader, the life breath,
> The fire of destruction, and the devoured offering (the moon).
> He is all that has been or shall be, eternal.
> Knowing him, one crosses beyond death.
> There is no other way to liberation (Kaivalya).[10]

Running through Śiva's historic variety of manifestations are some common motifs — that he embodies the five elements, has three eyes, is the source of internal bliss, and is the "lord of sleep." The lord of sleep designation is different from Viṣṇu, whose dream state is said to bring into existence our waking reality. Rather, Śiva's deep sleep is the one we all experience but never remember. In the yogic view, this deep-sleep state is the time we spend recharging with the numinous source, kind of like when we plug in our iPhone or BlackBerry at night. The reason that we never remember this period is that our conscious mind shuts down in order to get close to the highest self. If we were to develop our awareness to a state that we could remember this, we would be like the all-knowing, all-seeing source that is aware of all moments of time: Śiva.

Śiva is equipped for anything. His drum, the *ḍamaru,* which is shaped like two triangles whose points meet in the middle, is a symbol of the rhythms that bring all manifestation into being.[11] He carries a trident, whose three points represent each of the three qualities of the universe (*guṇa*), over which he has mastery. He stands on a tiger's pelt as a symbol of his power over nature. He's rumored to have slain the tiger when he was thrown into a pit by a couple of jealous sages whose wives thought he was quite a good-looking dude. And he has three eyes. Apparently, one day, in a playful mood, Pārvatī came up behind Śiva and covered his eyes, saying, "Guess who?" But Śiva couldn't see anything. In order to be able to continue to see all of creation, he manifested a third eye in the middle of his forehead. He then guessed correctly that it was Pārvatī standing behind him. Finally, Śiva is cloaked in ash (the sacred *vibhūti* of the fire ceremony), has dreadlocked hair (in which the crescent moon is nestled), and is covered in cobras because he is beyond the fear of death.[12]

Śiva's Magic Number Five

Śiva is the original yogi. All forms of the practice come from his initial realization of yoga on top of Mount Kailāsa. He's the original yoga teacher, and his teachings are contained within the cave of the heart (*hṛdayam*) in his form as Maheśvara. We find these hidden teachings within us through yoga practices, but particularly through the power of sound and speech, over which Śiva also has dominion. In his form as the lord of the dance (Nāṭarāja), the rhythm of his *ḍamaru* brings about existence itself, and "the process of the manifestation of thought into speech is equated with the process of cosmic manifestation through which Śiva gives birth to the universe."[13] And much of creation is grouped into fives, which we see reflected throughout Śiva's aspects and the elements of the universe: earth, fire, wind, water, and ether. The manifestation of thought into speech is reflected in Śiva's five-fold components, which are akin to the five *kośa* (or sheaths; for a description, see the Gāyatrī Mantra, page 65).

First, we have Śiva as the conqueror of death. This is the moment of silence. When one knows oneself to be deathless, then the source of all things is found, and silence is the expression. There is utter peace and joy in this form of Śiva, known as the liberator, or *mṛtyuṁjaya* (see the Oṁ Tryambakaṁ mantra, page 103), and so it is associated with *ānandamaya kośa*. Second is the image of Dakṣiṇāmūrti, the south-facing god who faces the flow of the light from the sun, which is the carrier of the knowledge of the intellect (*buddhi*). This image is depicted atop the rhythm of the letters of the mantra because "to take form, knowledge will depend upon the device of language. The word is the manifested form of knowledge."[14] And so Dakṣiṇāmūrti is associated with the *vijñānamaya kośa*. When knowledge turns into thinking and ambition, then words begin to express desire and attachment. The form of Śiva embodied here is known as Kāmeśvara, or the "lord of lust." This desirous aspect is dominated by the five senses, which are ever-present in the *manomaya kośa* as our mental energy turns outward. When life expresses itself through the life force, *prāṇa*, which we feel as the breath (for more, see The Three Mahāvakyas mantra, page 111), Śiva appears as Paśupati, the great, benevolent lord of the world. *Prāṇa* is contained within the five vital energies (known as *prāṇavāyu*) of the *prāṇamaya kośa*, which give expression to our words, just as *prāṇa* gives expression to all forms of life. Finally, we see the ultimate manifestation both of being and language expressed in Śiva's fifth form, Bhūteśa. As the lord of the five elements, Bhūteśa embodies the physical layer of *annamaya kośa*. This aspect is mirrored in the ultimate expression of thought into speech (*vāk*). And there we have it — the five layers of Śiva, the five elements, the five expressions of thought into speech, and the five *kośa*.

But wait, there's more.

Śiva also has a five-faced expression, with four heads facing each of the cardinal directions, and one head facing the sky. It seems that Śiva is dominated by the number five, as well as by the power of sound. It's no wonder that everything he is said to embody can be felt and learned within the five-syllable mantra that invokes his essence: *namaḥ śivāya*.

So, Who Is This Śiva Guy, Anyway?

The ultimate yogi. The five-faced knower of all. The ash-covered meditating mendicant. The loyal husband of the ever-evolving Pārvatī. The dreadlocked deity whose popularity has survived since antiquity. Śiva is cool as a cucumber. It's no wonder that chanting his name and invoking his presence can confer unbelievable boons. The legendary sage Vyasa discovered this and realized the essential secret of life.

According to a story in the Śiva Purāṇa, the great sage Vyasa, who legend says wrote many of the sacred spiritual texts in the Vedic tradition (including the Mahābhārata, eighteen of the Upaniṣad, and compiled the Veda into four books), was locked in a state of constant meditation along the Sarasvatī River. He was doing his best to attain a state of enlightenment through enormous effort and penance. Another sage, Sanat Kumara, came flying in on a fancy chariot and asked Vyasa exactly what he was doing. Vyasa said, "Well, I'm trying to achieve the supreme knowledge of the numinous through intense meditation and ascetic practices. But it's really hard."

Sanat Kumara took pity on Vyasa. He'd been around the block and seen people work their tails off just to attain some modicum of spiritual evolution. It was difficult to watch people struggle and suffer along the spiritual path, so he offered some sagely advice.

"You know, Vyasa? There was a time that I did it the hard way, too. I thought that austere penance and crazy bouts of meditation would earn me cosmic chits toward peace and salvation. Not so, it just made me more tense and earnest in my striving. Eventually, I learned that the best way to finding a sense of freedom is through hearing and singing to Śiva. Through proper listening and mantra, all my delusions were destroyed, and I realized the power of *satchitananda*: being, consciousness, and bliss. It is the mere chanting of Śiva's name that allowed me to realize this."

Śiva's Ultimate Point: Following Bliss

Here's the simple truth. Enjoy life. Because this life is just too short for anything else. Śiva's different aspects and attitudes show us this. Sometimes he gets angry, so he makes up for it. He meditates, and then balances this by hanging out with his wife and two sons. He loves his cow, and he is always a little bit intoxicated by the nectar of the moon. He is cool as a cucumber and through his cool-headedness, he shows us how to be that way, too. His mantra, *namaḥ śivāya*, is a gateway to access that feeling, and to come to know our own *satchitananda* (*satcitānanda*), which is the blissful point of our existence. To follow our bliss is to lead a rich and wonderful life. Joseph Campbell explains it this way:

> The word "Sat" means being. "Chit" means consciousness. "Ananda" means bliss or rapture. I thought, "I don't know whether my consciousness is proper consciousness or not; I don't know whether what I know of my being is proper being or not; but I do know where my rapture is, so let

me hang on to rapture, and that will bring me both my consciousness and my being." I think it worked.[15]

No matter how we get there, the key to a life well lived is finding the source of our "rapture." Not crazy asceticism. Not spiritual hierarchy. Not dogma or doctrine. Not slaving away to fulfill any "should" or "should not." But, purely and simply, finding our bliss. Campbell hit on something when he translated this point for the Western mind. It's a concept that embodies the nature of yoga itself, which is pure bliss. And, remember, the nature of yoga is our true nature. It exists within us from the moment we come into this life and will be with us until the moment we exit this life. How do we find it?

We listen.

21. Oṁ Śāntiḥ

Every human being deserves peace, and every human being yearns for connection. It is connection that brings peace. When we connect to another and see ourselves as that other, we become peaceful toward those we encounter. This is the crux of what Gandhi meant when he famously said, "Be the change you wish to see in the world." Connection is the platform for internal transformation that allows us to project peace into our surroundings. With that in our minds and hearts, we traditionally end chants or spiritual practices with this chant, which asks for peace three times over:

ॐ शान्तिः शान्तिः शान्तिः ।
oṁ śāntiḥ śāntiḥ śāntiḥ
oṁ peace, peace, peace

Peace Within, Peace Without, Peace Everywhere

This threefold invocation of peace reflects the great trinities that consume our outer and inner world. We find triumvirates in all aspects of our life, in our mythologies and our psyche. In regards to our psyche, in childhood we first develop a strong sense of individual ego; then, as adults, we use our spiritual practice to undo the grasp of the ego; and finally, as a self-aware person, we attain the ability to look as an individual through the lens of the completely connected self. Indeed, this perspective radiates peace, as we understand that every being on earth looks out from the self-same window, and all desire freedom from suffering. In this way, we come to feel, know, and experience that we are all intimately connected.

As we chant *śāntiḥ śāntiḥ śāntiḥ*, we are requesting peace on every level possible, for ourselves, for others, and for the union of all. Where do we start? Do we work tirelessly to try and change the world outside of us? Or do we start within? While both methods have value and can create peace, the only sure method is starting within. Leo Tolstoy cleverly said, "Everyone thinks of changing the world, but no one thinks of changing himself." In fact, the only person we are guaranteed to be able to change is ourself! The only person to whom we can guarantee peace is ourself. If we are going to start, we have to start within. Peace of mind is contagious. When we fully possess it, it will radiate outward and effect the lives of those we encounter, no matter what good works we do. And good works remain largely pointless if we are internally disturbed, judgmental, or angry — disconnected from a life where what we do matters to others.

Might as well work with what we've got.

To this end, the spiritual practices of yoga help to shine us up like a new penny, ready to radiate peace. Because yoga always does its job. No matter what type of practice we prefer, or what teacher we learn from, the yoga will always do its job, rooting out the source of agitation and separation to reveal the state of stillness and peaceful connection. When we know peace, we can more easily bring it to others. Where do we find it? Within the solace of our own hearts. This is where peace is kept. Bred. Grown. Harvested to spread abundantly throughout our life. We release it by freeing ourselves of everything that is antithetical to peace — apathy, hurt, separation, and isolation. Transcending these binding qualities allows peace to reveal itself from within us. It then becomes a state of mind. Interestingly, the iconic poet T. S. Eliot ends his poem *The Waste Land* with the prayer *śāntiḥ śāntiḥ śāntiḥ*, and he translates *śāntiḥ* (*shanti*) as "the peace which passeth understanding." What lies beyond understanding, beyond the realm of thinking, is silence.

Peace brings us to silence. The stillness before movement shakes things up and orders and separates. Silence is the numinous source, and the meaning is given when sound arises. The word *silence* comes from the latin root *silere*, which means "to be still." May stillness bless our heart of hearts. May the peace of silence give rise to the music and meaning of our lives.

ॐ शान्तिः शान्तिः शान्तिः ।
oṁ śāntiḥ śāntiḥ śāntiḥ

Acknowledgments

I offer this book to readers with great gratitude and tremendous joy. However, it would not have been possible without the extraordinary help of some very gifted and talented people. First and foremost, I offer my thanks to my beloved agent, Michele Martin, and editorial director extraordinaire Georgia Hughes. These two are the charioteers at the helm, and I could not have gotten this far without their warmhearted guidance. The great editor Jeff Campbell worked like the dickens to make these words shine.

Many *pranam*s to Dr. John Casey for his help with the Sanskrit throughout this book. To my dearest friend and artistic master, Chris Yeazel, many thanks for his illustrative ability to bring to life the myths herein. To the lovely Emma Segal, I am tremendously grateful for her cover design, which is pure awesomeness.

Much gratitude to Tracy Cunningham for her design skills used to bring the art elements together, and to Tona Pearce Myers for the lovely layout. Thanks go to Kristen Cashman and Jonathan Wichmann for their help with editorial details and the finishing touches. This book's success is owed to the delightful work of Kim Corbin whose skipping spirit helped to create ripples of sacred sound.

Thanks are humbly given to the bright light Jyothi Chalam,

who generously shared with me the story about Lakṣmī on a hot summer day in Hong Kong. For planting the seeds, watching them sprout, and being there to offer support, I am grateful for Dave Stringer — his friendship and his foreword.

Because it takes a village to raise a book, I am indebted to my beloved Kaivalya Yoga Method crew, for whom I happily submitted myself to the mercy of the gods to create this book. Tremendous thanks go to Sweetleaf LIC, where warm drinks and smiles housed a second office, fueling my fervor for the written word. And to my dear friend Cara Ferrick and her charming family, I offer thanks for their support and encouragement from start to finish.

To my mother, who taught me how to sing and never let me give up, I give many thanks. And, finally, to my grandmother, whose first big lesson to me was "God lives in your heart."

I have been blessed by many who have supported me on this path — none of you are overlooked, and I thank you for all the ways in which you have held me up and allowed me to shine.

Endnotes

Introduction

1. For more about myth and the hero's journey, see my online e-course called "Following Bliss: A Modern Mystic's Guide to the Hero's Journey," which is available on my website, alannak.com.
2. Quotes by Candace S. Alcorta from "Music and the Miraculous: The Neurophysiology of Music's Emotive Meaning," in *Miracles: God, Science, and Psychology in the Paranormal*, ed. J. Harold Ellens, vol. 3, *Parapsychological Perspectives* (Westport, CT: Praeger, 2008), 230–52.
3. Joachim-Ernst Berendt, *The World Is Sound: Nada Brahma: Music and the Landscape of Consciousness* (Rochester, VT: Destiny, 1987), 119.

Part One: Classic Mantras

1. Joachim-Ernst Berendt, *The World Is Sound: Nada Brahma: Music and the Landscape of Consciousness* (Rochester, VT: Destiny, 1987), 132.
2. For more on the science of these vibrations, see S. W. Hawking, *A Brief History of Time: From the Big Bang to Black Holes* (Toronto: Bantam, 1988).
3. For more complete versions of the stories in this mantra on Brahmā and Viṣṇu, see Alanna Kaivalya and Arjuna van der Kooij, *Myths of the Asanas: The Stories at the Heart of the Yoga Tradition* (San Rafael, CA: Mandala, 2010).

4. I heard this from Yogi Narayana Baba and loved it. For more, visit www.narayanababa.com.
5. For one of the most cogent academic descriptions of Sāṁkhya philosophy, see Edwin F. Bryant and Patanjali, *The Yoga Sūtras of Patanjali: A New Edition, Translation, and Commentary with Insights from the Traditional Commentators* (New York: North Point, 2009).
6. For more on Mark Whitwell, visit www.heartofyoga.com.
7. Alain Daniélou, *The Myths and Gods of India: The Classic Work on Hindu Polytheism from the Princeton Bollingen Series* (Rochester, VT: Inner Traditions International, 1991), 125.
8. Joachim-Ernst Berendt, *The World Is Sound: Nada Brahma: Music and the Landscape of Consciousness* (Rochester, VT: Destiny, 1987), 41.
9. For a brief overview of the chakras, see Alanna Kaivalya and Arjuna van der Kooij, *Myths of the Asanas* (San Rafael, CA: Mandala Press, 2010).
10. The story of "The Knight of the Cart" appears in *Four Arthurian Romances* by Chretien de Troyes, written in the twelfth century.
11. For Hanuman's full story, see Alanna Kaivalya and Arjuna van der Kooij, *Myths of the Asanas* (San Rafael, CA: Mandala Press, 2010).
12. This notion is found throughout Joseph Campbell's works, but in particular, see Joseph Campbell, *The Masks of God: Primitive Mythology* (New York: Viking, 1959), 64.
13. Swami Prabhavananda, *The Upanishads: Breath of the Eternal* (Hollywood, CA: Vedanta Press, 1975), 180.
14. This translation is from Eknath Easwaran and Michael N. Nagler, *The Upanishads* (Petaluma, CA: Nilgiri, 1987).
15. Joachim-Ernst Berendt, *The World Is Sound: Nada Brahma: Music and the Landscape of Consciousness* (Rochester, VT: Destiny, 1987), 90.
16. This translation is from Eknath Easwaran and Michael N. Nagler, *The Upanishads* (Petaluma, CA: Nilgiri, 1987).
17. Ibid.
18. Ibid., 46.
19. Ibid.

20. Stephen Mitchell, *The Gospel According to Jesus: A New Translation and Guide to His Essential Teachings for Believers and Unbelievers* (New York: HarperCollins, 1991), 55.
21. For more on Śrī Brahmānanda Sarasvatī, visit anandaashram.org.

Part Two: Traditional Kirtans

1. For an example of modern-day kirtan, check out the music on my website, alannak.com. Chris Grosso and I perform as a two-piece kirtan band blending modern melodies with traditional chants. Oh, and Chris plays an all-American drum kit!
2. Find the story in Alanna Kaivalya and Arjuna van der Kooij, *Myths of the Asanas: The Stories at the Heart of the Yoga Tradition* (San Rafael, CA: Mandala, 2010).
3. Find this story in Alanna Kaivalya and Arjuna van der Kooij, *Myths of the Asanas: The Stories at the Heart of the Yoga Tradition* (San Rafael, CA: Mandala, 2010).
4. Robert Svoboda, *Aghora: At the Left Hand of God* (Albuquerque, NM: Brotherhood of Life, 1986), 98–101.
5. Elaine H. Pagels, *The Gnostic Gospels* (New York: Random House, 1979), 126.
6. Called the Prajṣāpāramitā Hṛdaya, or literally, "The Transcendant Wisdom of the Cave of the Heart." There are many fine translations of these simple teachings. Many can be found free online.
7. My favorite version of the Bhagavad Gītā with commentary is the three volume set by Eknath Easwaran, *The End of Sorrow, Like a Thousand Suns*, and *To Love Is to Know Me* (Tomales, CA: Nilgiri Press, 1979).
8. This story is told in Alanna Kaivalya and Arjuna van der Kooij, *Myths of the Asanas: The Stories at the Heart of the Yoga Tradition* (San Rafael, CA: Mandala, 2010).
9. Malcolm Gladwell, *Outliers: The Story of Success* (New York: Little, Brown and Company, 2008).
10. Alain Daniélou, *The Myths and Gods of India: The Classic Work on Hindu Polytheism from the Princeton Bollingen Series* (Rochester, VT: Inner Traditions International, 1991), 194.

11. Many of the details about Śiva here are from Daniélou, *The Myths and Gods of India*, 215, 218.
12. Find this story in Alanna Kaivalya and Arjuna van der Kooij, *Myths of the Asanas: The Stories at the Heart of the Yoga Tradition* (San Rafael, CA: Mandala, 2010).
13. Alain Daniélou, *The Myths and Gods of India: The Classic Work on Hindu Polytheism from the Princeton Bollingen Series* (Rochester, VT: Inner Traditions International, 1991), 206.
14. Ibid., 207.
15. Joseph Campbell, *The Hero with a Thousand Faces* (Princeton, NJ: Princeton University Press, 1968), 120.

Glossary

abhaya: the embodiment of fearlessness

adharma: unrighteousness or losing one's way

Ādiśeṣa (Adishesha): the great serpent

ahaṁkāra: personal ego or "I AM"-ness

ahata: struck

aiṁ: seed sound for Sarasvatī

ajapa: silent mantra repetition

amṛtam: nectar of immortality

anāhata: unstruck, also the name for the heart *cakra*

ānandamaya: the bliss layer of the body

Ananta: the serpent couch of Viṣṇu

annamaya: the food layer of the body

Arjuna: the great warrior from the Bhagavad Gītā

āsana: literally, "seat"; also, the common word for "posture" in modern-day yoga practice

aṣṭāṅga (*ashtanga*): the eight-limbed path described by Patañjali; also, the modern-day yoga practice popularized by Shri K. Pattabhi Jois

asura: demons

ātman: soul

avatāra (avatar): descended, human form of Viṣṇu

avidyā: ignorance, or literally, "absence of light"

Bhagavad Gītā (Bhagavad Gita): literally, "song of God"; spiritual text featuring dialogue between Kṛṣṇa and Arjuna

bhakta: one who practices bhakti yoga

bhakti: the yoga of devotion

bīja: seed, typically a one-syllable "seed" mantra, like *oṁ*

Brahmā: the four-faced creator god

Brahman: the numinous god, without quality and inexpressible

buddhi: enlightened consciousness

cakra (chakra): spinning wheel of energy (seven in the physical body)

Candra (Chandra): god of the moon

deva: god

devī: goddess

dhāraṇā: sixth limb of the *aṣṭāṅga* yoga practice, intense concentration

dharma: righteousness, or one's personal duty

Dhruva: the boy sage

dhyāna: seventh limb of the *aṣṭāṅga* yoga practice, focused meditation

Durgā: goddess of war

gaṁ: seed sound for Gaṇeśa

Gaṇapati: sweet name for Gaṇeśa

Gaṇeśa (Ganesh): elephant-headed god, known as remover of obstacles or revealer of possibilities

Gaṅga: goddess of the Ganges River in India

gāyatrī: name of a chant as well as a classic rhyming meter

graha: to be gripped by (for example, to be gripped by the power of the moon)

guṇa: quality, there are three distinct qualities (*guṇa*) of the universe

haṁsa: swan, the vehicle of Sarasvatī

Hanuman: the monkey god

haṭha: literally, "intense," also, "sun and moon"

iḍā: name of the left-sided energy channel in the body

Indra: lord of the heavens

indriya: organs of action, sensory organs

īśvara: personalized form of god

jīva: soul

Kailāsa (Kailash): mountain abode of Śiva

kaivalya: ultimate independence or freedom, synonym of enlightenment

Kālī: goddess of death

karma: action

kīrtana (kirtan): call-and-response chanting, participatory repetition of mantra with music

kośa (*kosha*): layer of the body

Kṛṣṇa (Krishna): *avatāra* of Viṣṇu; literally, "the all-attractive one"

kuṇḍalinī: a form of *śakti*, synonymous with consciousness

Lakṣmī (Lakshmi): goddess of abundance

līlā: the divine play

mahā: great

Mahābhārata: Indian epic tale of the war between two families

mahāyogi: great yogi; also feminine: *mahāyoginī*

māyā: veil of illusion made up of the *guṇa*

Maheśvara (Maheshvara): alternate name for Śiva; literally, "intense lord"

maṇḍala: design imparting the geometric nature of divinity

manomaya: the mind (emotional) layer of the body

mantra: uplifting phrase designed to elevate consciousness, usually in Sanskrit (*Saṁskṛta*)

moha: delusion

mokṣa (*moksha*): liberation from karmic bonds

mṛtyuṁjaya: liberation

mudrā: physical gesture to direct energy

nāda: sacred sound

nāḍī: energetic channel

namaḥ: name, to invoke a name is to invoke the name's essential quality

nāmarūpa: literally, "name is form"; the principle that the name of something is its form

Nārada: the cosmic minstrel

Nāṭarāja: the lord of the dance, an epithet for Śiva

oṁ: the expression of the fundamental cosmic vibration

paramātma: great soul or "over-soul"

Pārvatī: an aspect of Śakti, the consort of Śiva

Patañjali: author of the Yoga Sūtra

piṅgalā: name of the right-sided energy channel of the body

pradīpikā: to shed light on

prakṛti: manifest form

prāṇa: life force

prāṇamaya: the physiological layer of the body

prāṇaśakti (*prana shakti*): energy of the life force

praṇava: the name for *oṁ*; literally, "ever new"

prāṇāyāma: breath work, or the fourth limb of the *aṣṭāṅga yoga* path; literally, "restraint of the life force"

pūjā: ritual ceremony performed at an altar

pūrṇa: fullness or emptiness

puruṣa (*purusha*): the unmanifest reality, pure potential

puṣṭi (*pushti*): completely nourished or full

Rādhā: consort of Kṛṣṇa

rajas: the energetic *guṇa*

rākṣasa (*rakshasa*): demon

Rāma: *avatāra* of Viṣṇu, the great king of Ayodhya and hero of the Rāmāyana

Rāmāyana: the epic story of King Rāma

Rāvaṇa: the evil demon in the Rāmāyana

Rohiṇī: one of the Nakṣatra, consort of Candra

ṛṣi (*rishis*): ancient sages or seers who were said to have received the wisdom of the Veda and the language of Saṁskṛta

Rukmiṇī: wife of Kṛṣṇa

śabda (*shabda*): sacred sound, synonym of *nāda*

sahasra: seventh *cakra*; literally, "thousand-petaled lotus"

Śakti (Shakti): The goddess of universal energy

śakti (*shakti*): universal energy (typically feminine)

sama: same

samādhi: enlightenment, or the eighth limb of the *aṣṭāṅga yoga* path

Sāṁkhya: one of the "six views" of Indian philosophy, basis of yoga philosophy

saṁsāra: cycle of karma

Saṁskṛta (Sanskrit): literally, "perfectly made"

śaraṇaṁ (*sharanam*): refuge

Sarasvatī (Saraswati): goddess of arts, learning, and music

satsaṅga (*satsang*): gathering of like-minded individuals in pursuit of truth

sattva: the light *guṇa*

śava (*shava*): corpse

Savitṛ (Savitur): god who brings light

siddhi: yogic powers

śiṣya (*shishya*): student

Sītā: wife of King Rāma

Śiva (Shiva): god of destruction

Skanda: speedy brother of Gaṇeśa

śloka (*shloka*): phrase

soma: nectar of the moon

śraddhā (*shraddha*): faith, the contents of one's heart

Śrī (Shri): honorific term meaning "luminous"

śrūti (*shruti*): that which has been heard through sacred communication

śūnyatā (*shunyata*): emptiness

suṣumnā (*sushumnah*): ray of light, central *nāḍī*

sūtra: short aphorism; literally, "thread"

svāhā: a word of offering; literally, "I offer into the sacred fire"

tamas: the heavy *guṇa*

tapasya: fervent spiritual practice; literally, "to burn"

ujjāyī: victorious breath

Upaniṣad (Upanishads): sacred texts; literally, "to sit near"

vāk: voice or speech

Vasiṣṭha: great yogic sage

Veda (Vedas): oldest known spiritual texts; literally, "knowledge"

vijñānamaya: the intellectual layer of the body

vinyāsa: literally "to consciously place"; also a term used for modern-day yoga practice indicating breath and movement

Viṣṇu (Vishnu): god of preservation

viveka: perfect discernment

vṛtti: turning or whirling of both mind and breath

Yāma: god of death

yoga: literally, "union"; the word implies both the practice and the state of being united

yogi: one who is adept at yoga. In Sanskrit, masculine is *yogin*; feminine is *yoginī*.

Bibliography

Berendt, Joachim-Ernst. *The World Is Sound: Nada Brahma: Music and the Landscape of Consciousness*. Rochester, VT: Destiny, 1987.

Bryant, Edwin F., and Patanjali. *The Yoga Sūtras of Patanjali: A New Edition, Translation, and Commentary with Insights from the Traditional Commentators*. New York: North Point, 2009.

Buck, William. *Mahabharata*. Berkeley: University of California, 1973.

Campbell, Joseph. *The Hero with a Thousand Faces*. Princeton, NJ: Princeton University Press, 1968.

———. *The Masks of God: Primitive Mythology*. New York: Viking, 1959.

Campbell, Joseph, and Bill D. Moyers. *The Power of Myth*. New York: Doubleday, 1988.

Campbell, Joseph, and Diane K. Osbon. *A Joseph Campbell Companion: Reflections on the Art of Living*. New York: HarperCollins, 1991.

A Course in Miracles. Mill Valley, CA: Foundation for Inner Peace, 1975.

Daniélou, Alain. *The Myths and Gods of India: The Classic Work on Hindu Polytheism from the Princeton Bollingen Series*. Rochester, VT: Inner Traditions International, 1991.

Dimmitt, Cornelia. *Classical Hindu Mythology: A Reader in the Sanskrit Purāṇas*. Philadelphia: Temple University Press, 1978.

Easwaran, Eknath. *The End of Sorrow*. Petaluma, CA: Nilgiri, 1979.

———. *Like a Thousand Suns*. Petaluma, CA: Nilgiri, 1979.

———. *To Love Is to Know Me*. Petaluma, CA: Nilgiri, 1979.

Easwaran, Eknath, and Michael N. Nagler. *The Upanishads*. Petaluma, CA: Nilgiri, 1987.

Edinger, Edward F. *Ego and Archetype: Individuation and the Religious*

Function of the Psyche. New York: Putnam and the C. G. Jung Foundation for Analytical Psychology, 1972.

Gladwell, Malcolm. *Outliers: The Story of Success*. New York: Little, Brown and Company, 2008.

Hawking, S. W. *A Brief History of Time: From the Big Bang to Black Holes*. Toronto: Bantam, 1988.

Jacobi, Jolande. *Complex: Archetype; Symbol*. London: Routledge, 1959.

Jung, C. G. *Memories, Dreams, Reflections*. New York: Pantheon, 1963.

———. *Psychology and Religion*. New Haven, CT: Yale University Press, 1938.

———. *The Psychology of Kundalini Yoga*. Princeton, NJ: Princeton University Press, 1996.

Jung, C. G., and Anthony Storr. *The Essential Jung*. Princeton, NJ: Princeton University Press, 1983.

Jung, C. G., and Marie-Louise von Franz. *Man and His Symbols*. Garden City, NY: Doubleday, 1964.

Kaivalya, Alanna, and Arjuna van der Kooij. *Myths of the Asanas: The Stories at the Heart of the Yoga Tradition*. San Rafael, CA: Mandala, 2010.

Mitchell, Stephen. *The Gospel According to Jesus: A New Translation and Guide to His Essential Teachings for Believers and Unbelievers*. New York: HarperCollins, 1991.

Nietzsche, Friedrich Wilhelm. *Thus Spake Zarathustra*. New York: Heritage, 1967.

Pagels, Elaine H. *The Gnostic Gospels*. New York: Random House, 1979.

Śaṅkarācārya, T. K. V. Desikachar, and Kausthub Desikachar. *Ādi Śaṅkara's Yoga Tāravali:: English Translation and Commentary*. India: Krishnamacharya Yoga Mandiram, 2003.

Saraswati, Swami Chidanand. *Drops of Nectar Timeless Wisdom for Everyday Living*. N.p.: Wisdom Tree, 2007.

Svoboda, Robert. *Aghora: At the Left Hand of God*. Albuquerque, NM: Brotherhood of Life, 1986.

Williamson, Marianne. *A Return to Love: Reflections on the Principles of a Course in Miracles*. New York: HarperCollins, 1992.

Index

About the Author

Alanna Kaivalya, PhD, is the founder of The Kaivalya Yoga Method, offering a fresh take on yoga emphasizing the individual path while honoring tradition. Alanna has taught yoga since 2001 and began teaching and developing teacher trainings worldwide in 2003, including the online program YogaDownload. She received a PhD in mythological studies with an emphasis in depth psychology from Pacifica Graduate Institute. Her first book, *Myths of the Asanas*, showcased the myths behind the poses. She lives in New York City with Roxy the Wonderdog. Join her community at AlannaK.com.